L

NON-IN

DIABETES

© British Diabetic Association 1986, 1992

First published 1986 by Thorsons Publishing Group

This edition published 1992 by
Medikos Limited, Crowborough, England

A CIP catalogue record of this book
is available from the British Library

ISBN 0-9518787-0-0

Printed and bound by Embassy Press Limited
Crowborough, England

Living with
NON-INSULIN DEPENDENT
DIABETES

Dr. John L. Day M.D.,F.R.C.P.
Susan Brenchley B.Sc.,S.R.D.
Suzanne Redmond B.Sc.,R.G.N.

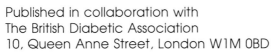
Published in collaboration with
The British Diabetic Association
10, Queen Anne Street, London W1M 0BD

MEDIKOS

Medikos Limited
Crowborough, England

Contents

Foreword

When I was first diagnosed with diabetes I was anxious and didn't know what to expect. I now know my fears were groundless and that people with diabetes *can* lead full and active lives once they understand their condition and how to control it.

I am therefore delighted to welcome this, the fully revised second edition of the British Diabetic Association Handbook. Prepared by diabetes experts, it contains all you need to know about non-insulin dependent diabetes, presented in an easy-to-read format. It is copiously illustrated and clearly and sympathetically written, so that even *I* can understand the most complex aspects of diabetes and its control!

The BDA Handbook is, of course, an invaluable reference book, but it is also an essential practical guide to living with diabetes. Nobody with diabetes should be without a copy.

Harry Secombe

Sir Harry Secombe CBE

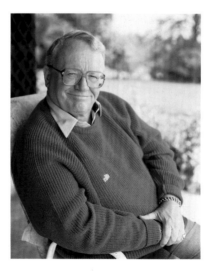

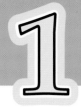

About diabetes

The purpose of this book

Fig. 1.1
The estimated numbers of people with diabetes

Diabetes or, to give it its full name, diabetes mellitus, is very common. In the United Kingdom there are more than 750,000 people with diabetes, of whom over 18,000 are children. Worldwide there are over 30 million known cases.

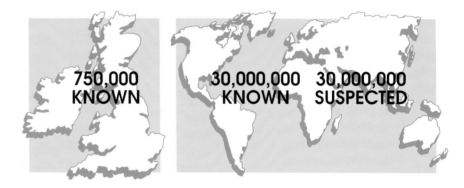

Although diabetes cannot be cured, it is hoped that you will come to recognize that there are steps you can take that will ensure that the effects on your life are kept to a minimum. We hope that the information given in this book will also allow you to discuss your diabetes and its effects freely and without embarrassment with your friends, relatives, or colleagues. You may wish to know about the causes of diabetes and so avoid undue worry that it is your or somebody else's fault. Our aim is to encourage you to follow the recommended treatment with optimism, to share your concerns with those available to help, and also to attend regularly for the medical checks which are necessary from time to time.

We assume that either you already know that you have diabetes, or are finding out more to help a relative or friend. It is not expected that you will read the book from cover to cover, but you may wish just to check on certain details or remind yourself of things that you may have learnt. The chapters have been divided with these possibilities in mind.

What is diabetes?

Diabetes is a disorder in which the mechanism for converting sugar (glucose) to energy is no longer functioning properly. This causes an abnormally high level of sugar in the blood and may give rise to a variety of symptoms. If the sugar levels remain high over several years, damage may be caused to various parts of the body. Treatment of diabetes is designed not only to **reverse** any symptoms but also to **prevent** any serious problems developing later.

How does diabetes develop?

Normally, the amount of sugar in the body is very carefully controlled. We obtain sugar from the food we eat, either from sweet things or from starchy foods (carbohydrates), such as bread and potatoes. Sugar can also be made by breaking down the body stores of starch in the liver. This will occur when the body needs an extra supply of sugar, for example after missing several meals, or following an injury, or during an illness.

The use of sugar to provide energy requires the presence of the hormone insulin. Insulin is released as the blood sugar rises after a meal. Its function is to return the sugar concentration to its original level. Less insulin is produced when the sugar level falls, for example during exercise. Insulin plays a vital role in maintaining the correct level of blood sugar.

When there is a shortage of insulin, or if the available insulin does not function correctly, then the blood sugar rises and diabetes results.

Fig. 1.2
Insulin rising and falling in response to the blood sugar
This shows the blood sugar rising after each meal or snack. This rise stimulates the release of insulin. The insulin returns the sugar level to normal.

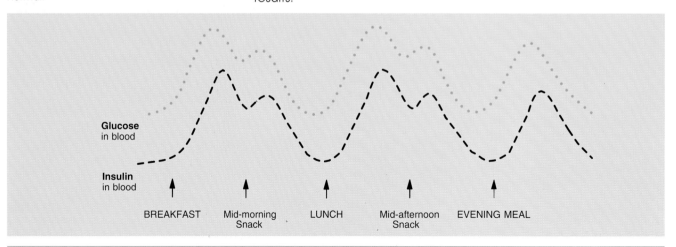

The normal range of blood sugar levels of someone who does not have diabetes is between 3.5 and 7.8 mmol/l.

A little history

Diabetes cannot be called a 'modern' disease. It has been referred to in ancient Egyptian, Indian, Roman, Japanese, and Chinese writings.

However, it was not until the last century that any significant advance was made in understanding the nature of diabetes. The first major breakthrough came in 1889. Two German scientists discovered that the removal of the pancreas, a large gland in the abdomen, gave rise to diabetes. It was also discovered that damage to clusters of cells in the pancreas, called islets of Langerhans, produced certain forms of diabetes, but it was not until 1921 that two Canadians, Frederick Banting and Charles Best, made their famous discovery of insulin.

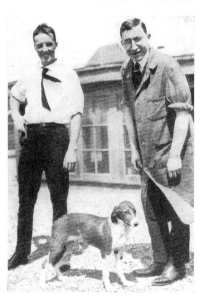

Fig. 1.3
Banting and Best

Frederick Banting and Charles Best, whose research led to the isolation of insulin. The photograph shows them with their famous dog, Marjorie, who was kept alive by insulin after her pancreas had been removed.

Who gets diabetes and the possible causes

In the United Kingdom, as many as one to two per 100 of the population and perhaps one in every 600 schoolchildren have diabetes. It can occur at any age, but is very rare in infants. It becomes common as people approach middle-age and in more elderly people.

There are two main types of diabetes.

1. **Non-insulin dependent diabetes** – sometimes called Type II diabetes or maturity onset diabetes.
2. **Insulin dependent diabetes** – sometimes called Type I diabetes or juvenile diabetes.

Non-insulin dependent diabetes

Cause

If you have non-insulin dependent diabetes you are still producing insulin, but it is either not being made in sufficient quantities or not working properly. **You do not need to take insulin in order to survive**. Most people with non-insulin dependent diabetes can be effectively treated by diet, or by a combination of diet and tablets. Sometimes, insulin injections may be necessary to establish perfect control of blood sugar levels. Despite continuing research the cause is not yet known.

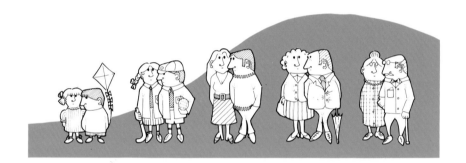

Who gets it?

Non-insulin dependent diabetes used to be called 'maturity onset diabetes'. This was because it mainly occurs in the middle and older age groups, although it can sometimes occur in young people. Overweight people are particularly likely to develop this type of diabetes. It tends to run in families, and it is slightly more common in women than men.

Insulin dependent diabetes

Cause

In this type of diabetes there is a complete or near complete absence of insulin, due to the destruction of the insulin-producing cells. With this type of diabetes **it is essential to have insulin treatment to survive.**

The exact cause of the damage to the insulin-producing cells is not known for certain, but a combination of factors may be involved including

● Damage to the insulin-producing cells by viral or other infections
● An abnormal reaction of the body against the insulin-producing cells.

Who gets it?

In general, it affects younger people (under 30 years of age), but occasionally it occurs in older age groups, even the very old. Both sexes are equally affected.

There is some tendency for insulin dependent diabetes to run in families, but the condition is far from being entirely inherited.

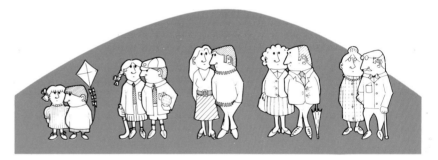

Other causes of diabetes

Diseases of the pancreas

A very few cases of diabetes are due to various diseases of the pancreas. These include inflammation (pancreatitis), or unusual deposits of iron. Mumps may sometimes have the same effect.

Accidents or illness

Major accidents or illnesses do not cause diabetes. However, they do sometimes produce a temporary increase in blood sugar.

If your diabetes was discovered during the course of an illness, it is most likely that you already had diabetes (even though you may not have had any symptoms). Some forms of hormone imbalance may also produce temporary diabetes.

Tablets

Some tablets can increase the blood sugar and reveal pre-existing diabetes. Steroid drugs, or water tablets (diuretics) which eliminate fluid from the body, may do this.

The contraceptive pill

This does not cause diabetes, but it may raise the blood sugar slightly in those already affected.

Heredity

If one parent has diabetes, his or her children are slightly more likely to develop diabetes than children in those families where no members are affected. Risks, however, are small. For example, the chances of developing diabetes before the age of 20 are perhaps only one in 100. Rarely, both parents have diabetes, in which case the chances are increased.

Non-insulin dependent diabetes is more commonly inherited than insulin dependent diabetes. However, this usually occurs in people who are middle aged or older and therefore their children are not usually affected until later in life. Diabetes is even more likely to develop if such children become overweight when they are middle-aged.

To summarize, it is possible for someone to inherit a tendency to diabetes, but **not** the condition itself. This only develops because of some other influence. Thus, there are very many people who never develop diabetes, even though they may have a strong family history of the disorder.

Symptoms and their severity

The main symptoms of diabetes are

- Extreme thirst and a dry mouth
- Passing large amounts of urine
- Weight loss
- Tiredness
- Itching of the genital organs
- Blurring of vision.

Non-insulin dependent diabetes

The symptoms develop over several weeks or months. **Diabetic coma does not occur in this type of diabetes.**

Some people fail to notice any symptoms, but after being treated they usually have more energy and feel considerably better. **Unfortunately, the presence of symptoms is no guide to the level of sugar in the blood, and it is essential that diabetes is treated, even when there are no symptoms.**

Symptoms are more likely to develop during another illness, such as a chest or urinary infection. This is because illness increases the blood sugar levels. The higher the blood sugar levels, the more obvious the symptoms of diabetes become.

Insulin dependent diabetes

Symptoms similar to those in non-insulin dependent diabetes tend to develop rather more quickly, over a few days or weeks. Without insulin treatment the condition progressively worsens, resulting in a significant weight loss, dehydration, vomiting, and the onset of drowsiness and diabetic coma. All these symptoms rapidly resolve with treatment.

Treatment

Diabetes is a very common disorder. **Although no 'cure' is possible, all types of diabetes can be treated and normal health restored.**

Treatment is with

● **Diet, or diet and tablets** – for non-insulin dependent diabetes.

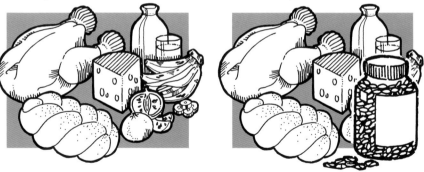

● **Insulin and diet** – for insulin dependent diabetes

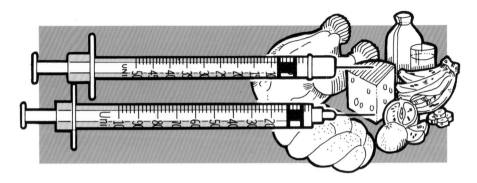

Treatment **must** be maintained throughout life. This is necessary not only to avoid symptoms, but also to minimize the risks of any later complications.

Both forms of treatment require some modification to daily routines, and the performance of checks to ensure that treatment is effective. However, you should be able to achieve these with only minimal disturbance to your daily life.

From Chapter 2 onwards, this Handbook explains in detail what has gone wrong in your type of diabetes and describes how, with correct treatment, you should be able to maintain effective control.

Modern treatment allows many thousands of people with diabetes to achieve complete, fruitful, healthy lives and to fulfil ambitions in all walks of life. Diabetes should not interfere with the vast majority of occupations. People with diabetes are found amongst our most successful actors, actresses, entertainers, politicians, first class footballers, sportsmen and women, and in all the professions. They bear witness to the fact that effective treatment can be combined with the highest achievement.

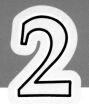

2 Non-insulin dependent diabetes

If you are fully to understand your treatment you will require some more information about this type of diabetes. The objectives of this chapter are to help you appreciate

- What has happened
- Why it may have occurred
- The explanation of any symptoms you may have experienced
- Why treatment is necessary, even if you have had no symptoms
- Why treatment must be continued.

So what happens when you develop diabetes?

In Chapter 1 the role of sugar control in the development of diabetes was briefly considered. To understand this further it is necessary to know some facts about the food you eat. This is made up of three basic types (Fig. 2.1) – carbohydrates, fats, and proteins, all of which are essential for a balanced diet. These three types of food are broken down by digestive processes in the intestine. The breakdown products of digestion are then absorbed into the bloodstream and carried to the individual body cells. Carbohydrates, found in starchy foods, such as bread and potatoes, are broken down and converted to sugar (glucose). Fat is converted to fatty acids and these and the glucose are used to provide energy in the body. When protein is digested the resulting amino acids are used to build cells and tissues. Any excess, however, is converted to glucose.

Fig. 2.1
Fats, carbohydrates, and proteins are essential for a balanced diet

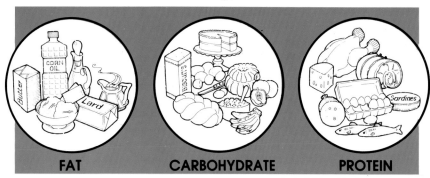

FAT   **CARBOHYDRATE**   **PROTEIN**

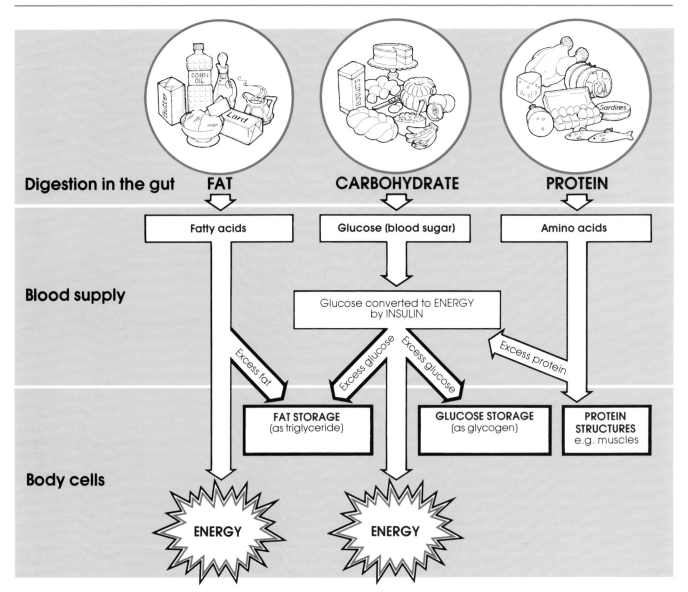

Digestion in the gut FAT CARBOHYDRATE PROTEIN

Fatty acids   Glucose (blood sugar)   Amino acids

Blood supply

Glucose converted to ENERGY
by INSULIN

Excess fat   Excess glucose   Excess glucose   Excess protein

FAT STORAGE
(as triglyceride)

GLUCOSE STORAGE
(as glycogen)

PROTEIN
STRUCTURES
e.g. muscles

Body cells

ENERGY   ENERGY

Fig. 2.2
Normal metabolism
In the presence of insulin, glucose can be converted to energy.

Where does blood sugar come from?

In the healthy individual, the level of blood sugar is kept within close limits. The major source of sugar is the food we eat. Blood sugar therefore goes up after a meal and falls when we are fasting. The main sources of blood sugar in food are

- **Sweet things**, e.g. sugar added to cereals, drinks, sweets, jams, etc.
- **Starchy foods**, e.g. bread, potatoes, cereals, flour, etc.
- **Other foods**, e.g. protein may be converted to glucose.

If sugar intake is more than the body requires, the excess is stored in the liver (Fig. 2.2). This store acts as a reserve for times of need, illness, or injury. But once liver stores are filled, any excess is converted to fat. This is what happens if you eat too much over a long period. Too much of the other fuels (fats and proteins) will ultimately have the same effect – both blood sugar and body weight will increase.

The importance of insulin

Insulin is the key to the conversion of sugar to energy, or its storage. It also helps to maintain the amount of stored energy by stopping excessive breakdown of fat. Insulin is produced by the pancreas, a gland situated at the back of the abdomen (Fig. 2.3).

The pancreas is able to sense the level of blood sugar. As the sugar level rises, the pancreas will release more insulin into the circulation (Fig. 2.4). This insulin reduces the blood sugar to the level at which it started. Thus, as the sugar level rises after a meal, the level of insulin increases as well. The level of insulin is therefore highest an hour or so following food, after which it falls back to its pre-meal level. The amount of insulin in the blood is lowest when you have not eaten, for example overnight.

When you are not eating, your blood sugar is kept steady and prevented from falling too low by a regular trickle of sugar into the blood from the body stores. This is finely balanced by a slow output of insulin. During exercise more sugar is used up, so in order to stop the level from falling too low, more sugar may be released from stores. The insulin level is reduced.

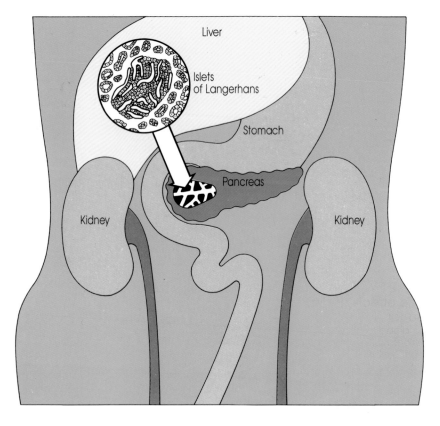

Fig. 2.3
The pancreas
The pancreas is a large gland positioned behind the stomach. It contains many cells which produce insulin. These are collected in clusters called islets of Langerhans.

At times of stress or injury more energy is required by the body and more sugar is produced, even if you are not eating. This sugar is then converted to energy by a slow release of insulin. The rise of blood sugar under these circumstances is controlled.

In your type of diabetes you are producing insulin, but not as much as you need (Fig. 2.5). The situation is made worse if you are overweight, because the amount of fat in the body interferes with the action of the insulin. The rise in blood sugar after a meal is greater than normal and it does not return as quickly to its pre-meal level. When not eating, the blood sugar also tends to creep up as the energy stores release sugar in an uncontrolled way.

Fig. 2.4
The control of blood sugar by insulin

Insulin released from the pancreas makes the blood sugar level fall. After 2–3 hours it returns to the same level as before the meal.

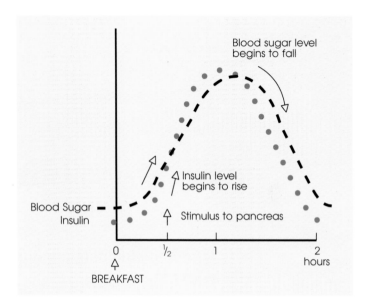

Fig. 2.5
The effects of diabetes on blood sugar

In diabetes, insufficient insulin results in an excessively high blood sugar. It does not return to the normal level after eating.

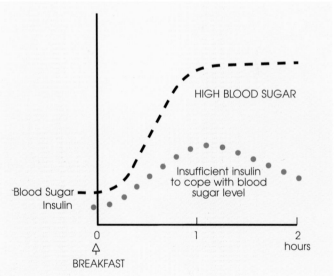

Fig. 2.6
Blood sugar levels
When the sugar reaches a certain level, it spills over into the urine. This level is called the 'renal threshold'.

As the blood sugar rises above normal, there comes a point when it begins to spill over into the urine.

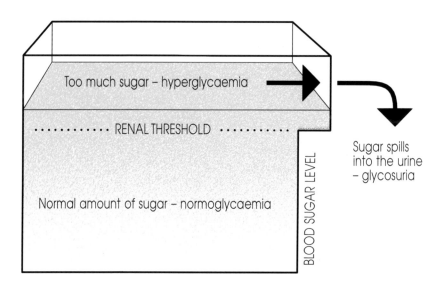

Usually, no sugar appears in the urine, so that when it is found it suggests that the blood sugar is too high. However, there are some people who spill sugar into the urine too easily, so that sugar appears in the urine but the blood sugar remains normal. This is called a 'low renal threshold'. In the case of diabetes, the presence of sugar in the urine means the blood sugar is too high.

Who gets diabetes and why?

There may be two factors which contribute to the development of your diabetes.

1. The pancreas may be unable to produce enough insulin to maintain the blood sugar within the normal range.
2. The pancreas may produce enough insulin, but it does not work effectively.

Non-insulin dependent diabetes occurs in various groups of individuals.

- It occurs most commonly in people who are overweight. Fat tissue interferes with the action of insulin, so that overweight people need considerably more insulin than normal individuals. If, in addition, an overweight person has a **lower than normal** production of insulin, because of a defect in the pancreas, the supply of insulin will be insufficient to control the blood sugar. Overweight people tend to eat more than their body needs, and their food provides more sugar than can be processed by the available insulin. In most cases, this type of diabetes can be readily controlled by simply eating less and losing weight, thereby allowing the insulin to work more effectively.
- This type of diabetes also occurs in people who are not overweight but who produce inadequate amounts of insulin.
- Some people at times of stress show a tendency to be unable to produce enough insulin. This tendency may only become obvious at times when more sugar than normal is required, such as during an illness or after injury. It is important to point out that injury or illness are not believed to cause diabetes, but rather that they make it more obvious.
- In some families there is a strong hereditary element, and diabetes may be passed from generation to generation. However, it is not inevitable.
- It appears to be more common in some parts of the world, such as South America or Malta, than in others, such as Alaska.

Symptoms of high blood sugar

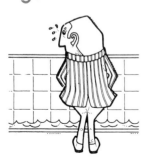

Sugar in the urine

As shown on page 14, one of the key features of a high blood sugar is spillage of sugar into the urine. This gives rise to three of the commonest symptoms of diabetes.

- **Passing large quantities of urine**

    In order to get rid of the excess sugar, more water is excreted by the kidneys. This results in the frequent passing of large volumes of urine, which may cause bed-wetting in some children, or incontinence in the elderly.

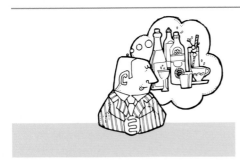

● Thirst

Because more water is leaving the body, the mouth becomes dry and thirst develops. This feeling may be very intense and disagreeable, and sometimes even talking and swallowing become difficult. Soft drinks which contain a lot of sugar should be avoided, as they actually increase the blood sugar, resulting in an even greater thirst.

● Genital soreness

When a large quantity of sugar is passed in the urine, it tends to cause irritation around the genital area. The infection called thrush may develop. Thrush frequently causes itching of the vulva in women and, less often, itching of the penis in men.

Breakdown of body energy stores

Because a shortage of insulin means that the blood sugar cannot be converted into energy, energy must be provided from elsewhere. Consequently, there is a breakdown of fat and protein with the following results.

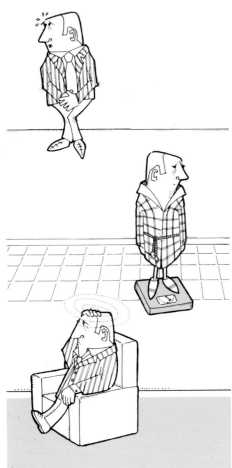

● Weight loss

Diabetes is one of the commonest causes of weight loss. In most people with diabetes this occurs at the onset of the disorder, and it ranges from a few pounds to 2–3 stones. Appetite is commonly unaffected and may even be increased. Not everyone loses weight, so do not ignore other symptoms.

● Tiredness and weakness

Tiredness, often accompanied by a sensation of weakness, is very common in uncontrolled diabetes. Some people find that they are more than usually prone to fall asleep at odd times, while others just feel they are growing old before their time. These symptoms can be readily reversed by treatment. Many people feel rejuvenated after treatment, even when they had previously been unaware of any abnormalities.

ALL THESE SYMPTOMS SHOULD DISAPPEAR SOON AFTER TREATMENT IS STARTED

If symptoms return, the sugar levels will have risen to too high a level and treatment will need to be adjusted.

Other effects of high blood sugar

● **Blurring of vision**

A high level of sugar in the body causes the lens of the eye to change slightly in shape, which may cause some blurring of vision. Sometimes this occurs after treatment has started. As the blood sugar returns to normal the lens may change shape again. These changes are only temporary, and the ability to focus should return to normal within a few weeks. **Therefore, it is wise not to have your eyes tested for at least two months after proper stabilization of your diabetes.**

● **Excessive loss of fluid/diabetic coma**

It is important to stress that in your type of diabetes, the so-called 'diabetic coma', which results from an extremely high blood sugar level, does not occur. During a vomiting illness, such as gastroenteritis, the blood sugar level may become unusually high. This can cause a significant increase in fluid loss.

Symptomless diabetes

Why treatment must be continued

Most people with diabetes are aware of symptoms when the blood sugar is very high. Others may be quite unaware of their condition. For instance, diabetes is often detected at a routine medical examination for insurance or employment purposes, or during an investigation of some quite unrelated illness.

● **Very often symptoms disappear during the early stages of treatment, even though the blood sugar is still above normal.**

● **You will need to learn how to check that your sugar levels are not too high, even if you have no symptoms.**

● **If your tests are too high, your treatment may need to be increased.**

● **Either way, treatment must be continued whether you have symptoms or not.**

Long-term effects of high blood sugar

If the blood sugar remains high for a period of years – even if it is not causing symptoms – it may cause harm. In particular, damage to the small blood vessels or nerves in the feet, the back of the eye, or the lens of the eye may occur. Early, effective treatment of diabetes should prevent this damage from developing. Occasionally, some of these problems may be present when your diabetes is first discovered. However, treatment for your diabetes should stop them from developing further. Complications of diabetes are considered in more detail in Chapter 7.

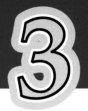

Diet treatment

This chapter describes the steps you need to take to control your diabetes and, in particular, gives details of the type of food you should eat.

There are two main aims of treatment

1. Eliminate symptoms

A high blood sugar level is largely responsible for your symptoms. The first aim of treatment is to reverse these by returning the blood sugar level to normal. Once treatment has started, your symptoms should disappear and should not recur if treatment is continued.

2. Prevent late complications

If a high blood sugar persists for many years, then the eyes, kidneys, and small nerves to the feet may be damaged. Therefore, there is every reason to **achieve normal blood sugars** and, by keeping to your treatment, reduce the risk of these complications.

People with diabetes are slightly more likely to develop problems with their major arteries, and this may lead to heart and leg trouble. This can be kept to a minimum by adjusting the diet in the way described below.

IT IS IMPORTANT THAT YOU CONTINUE WITH YOUR TREATMENT, EVEN WHEN THE SYMPTOMS HAVE GONE, AND THAT YOU UNDERGO REGULAR CHECKS TO ENSURE THAT YOUR CONTROL IS BEING MAINTAINED.

The steps you need to take

Adjust what you eat
- ● **Eat regular meals**
- ● **Reduce your weight**

  Most people with non-insulin dependent diabetes are overweight. Being overweight makes the insulin you produce less efficient. The most important measure needed to control blood sugar levels is to reduce weight. Your aim should be to reach your target weight, when the insulin you produce will be able to maintain your blood sugar at a normal level.

- ● **Control your sugar intake**

  It is important to avoid or reduce the amount of foods eaten which lead to a rapid rise in blood sugar, particularly sweets, sweetened drinks, and sugary puddings.

- ● **Reduce the amount of fat and fatty foods you eat**
- ● **Increase your intake of high-fibre foods**
- ● **Drink alcohol only in moderation**

All of these essential adjustments to your diet can be achieved fairly easily with time. You will still be able to eat interesting and pleasant food.

Exercise

If you are able, it is important that you should take regular exercise. This will not only help to keep your blood sugar down but, if necessary, will also help you reduce your weight.

Other treatment measures
- ● **Tablets**

  If the above measures prove inadequate, you may be advised to take some special tablets. These are not, however, a substitute for diet.

- ● **Insulin treatment**

  Insulin injections are only required when all the above measures have proved unsuccessful.

This chapter describes the changes you may need to make in the type of foods you eat.

Tablet and insulin treatment are described in subsequent chapters.

What will the diet be like?

The diet for diabetes is not a special diet as such. It is, in fact, a healthy way of eating, which can be recommended for everyone. The purpose of this section is to help you make the best choice in the food that you eat.

- Firstly, you may need to alter the **sort** of food you eat. Some foods should be restricted, some eaten only in moderation, and some may be eaten freely.
- Secondly, you may need to adjust the **amount** of food you eat, especially if you are overweight.

Food plays a very important part in our lives and therefore making changes to our diet can affect more than just meal times. Our eating patterns and the types of food we eat are often a lifelong habit. These habits are difficult to break, so do not expect to change your diet overnight. Look realistically at what you are eating and decide what changes could easily be made. Tackle these first and then go onto the rest.

The basic components of food

Our food is made up of three basic nutrients – carbohydrate, protein and fat. They are all essential for a balanced diet. Most foods contain mixtures of one or more of these nutrients. For example, milk contains carbohydrate, protein, and fat; eggs contain fat and protein; and pastry is mainly fat and carbohydrate. In general, vegetables and fruit contain little or no fat, while cheese, margarine, and meat contain no carbohydrate.

What are calories?

Calories are a measure of the amount of energy provided by the food you eat. Their official name is actually kilocalories (kcal), but they are usually referred to simply as calories. The term calorie has been used throughout this book.

All food provides calories, but some foods are more concentrated in calories than others. For example, a 100 g (4 oz) apple would provide you with around 50 calories, whereas 100 g (4 oz) of cheddar cheese would provide 400 calories. This is because every food contains different proportions of fat, carbohydrate, and protein. Fat contains twice as many calories, weight for weight, as either carbohydrate or protein. Therefore, those foods which have a high percentage of fat are likely to be highest in calories.

On food labels, the calorie value of a food is usually written as kcal/100 g. For example, if a label states 324 kcals/100 g, it means that a 100 g (4 oz) portion of the food would provide 324 calories. Sometimes you may come across the term kilojoule (kj). This is another way of describing the amount of energy in food.

If you take in more energy from food than you use on day-to-day activities, your weight will increase. If less, your weight will fall.

It is not necessary to count calories. However, if you are trying to lose weight, you may find it helpful to be aware of which foods are particularly high in calories.

Important components of the diet

Carbohydrate

Sugary and starchy foods are all sources of carbohydrate. All carbohydrates are broken down in the body to sugar, and so will cause the blood sugar level to rise. However, although all carbohydrate foods are eventually turned into sugar, eating high fibre starchy foods is encouraged, whereas eating sugary foods is not.

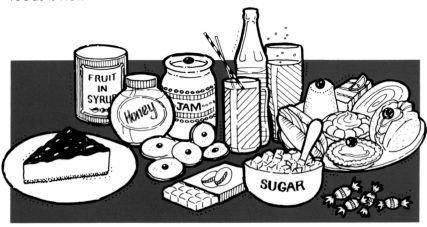

Fig 3.1
Carbohydrate: some typical foods containing large amounts of sugar

This is because starchy foods tend to be more slowly digested than sugary foods and so cause a slower, more controlled rise in the blood sugar level. At least half of your daily calories should come from starchy foods, e.g. bread, potatoes, pasta, and pulses.

Fig. 3.2
Carbohydrate: some typical starch
containing foods

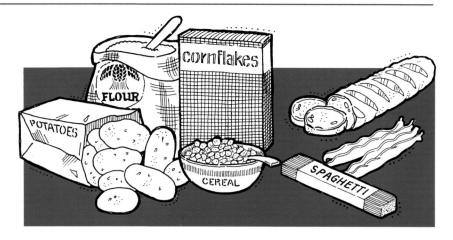

Fibre

Dietary fibre is a substance of plant origin which is not broken down in the human digestive system. Fruits and vegetables, and the outside coats of grains and cereals all contain dietary fibre. Starchy foods which are high in carbohydrate are usually good sources of fibre.

● **Soluble** fibre is the type of fibre found in oats, pulses (i.e. peas, beans, and lentils), and some fruit (Fig. 3.3).

● **Insoluble** fibre is the fibre found in wheat bran, wholemeal flour, wholemeal bread, brown pasta, and rice (Fig. 3.4).

High fibre foods tend to be bulky, so they fill you up more quickly. This is especially important if you are trying to lose weight.

Foods high in soluble fibre, such as peas, beans, oats, and lentils, have an especially good effect on diabetes control. They slow down the rise in blood sugar level after a meal, and they also help control the levels of fat in the blood.

Evidence also suggests that eating a diet containing lots of high fibre carbohydrate foods may help prevent constipation and diverticulitis (a disorder affecting the large intestine).

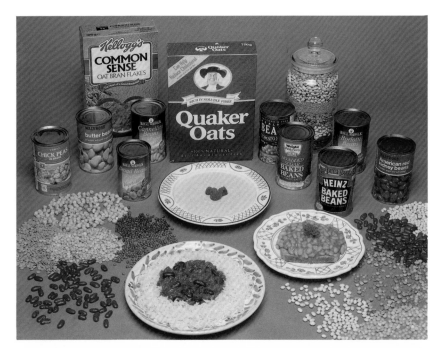

Fig. 3.3
Foods high in soluble fibre

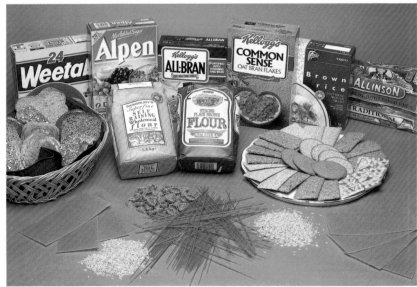

Fig. 3.4
Foods high in insoluble fibre

Protein

Foods high in protein include meat, milk, eggs, fish, dairy products, and pulses. Protein is essential in the diet, because it provides the building materials for the cells and tissues of the body. You will need to remember that foods high in protein also tend to be high in fat and therefore calories.

Fig. 3.5
Typical foods high in protein

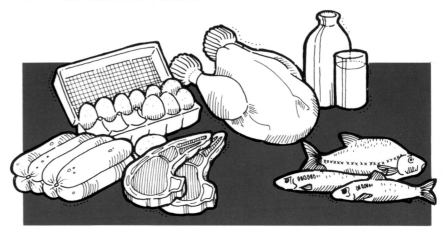

Fat

Obvious sources of fat are butter, margarine, oil, lard, and dripping; fatty meats and dairy products contain fat, too. You should also watch out for the fat found in cakes and pastries. Because even small amounts of fat contain a large number of calories, the fat content of the diet should be strictly controlled when losing weight. Only small quantities are necessary for good health.

There are three types of fat

● Saturated fats
● Polyunsaturated fats
● Monounsaturated fats.

They all contain the same amount of calories, but **saturated fats** particularly can raise blood cholesterol levels. Saturated fats are usually found in animal products, e.g. fatty meat, suet, lard, butter, cheese, full fat milk, and other dairy products.

Fig. 3.6
Common foods high in fat

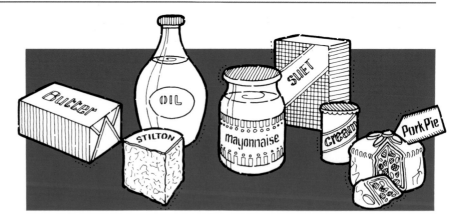

Foods high in **polyunsaturated fats** should be used in preference to foods high in saturated fats. The fat in oily fish, such as herring, tuna, and mackerel is largely of the polyunsaturated type. When choosing a cooking oil, pick sunflower, corn, or soya oil in preference to lard or dripping. Some vegetable oils are polyunsaturated, but many are not. Select those which state on the label that they are high in polyunsaturated fats.

Monounsaturated fats are found in olive and rapeseed oil and, like polyunsaturated fats, are preferable to saturated fats.

It is not the amount of **cholesterol** in the food which affects blood cholesterol. Most cholesterol in the body is made from other food, especially that which is high in saturated fats. Levels rise as you become overweight, so weight reduction not only helps your blood sugar but also your blood cholesterol.

IT IS IMPORTANT TO REMEMBER THAT ALL TYPES OF FAT ARE HIGH IN CALORIES AND ONLY SMALL QUANTITIES SHOULD BE USED. WHENEVER POSSIBLE, TRY TO CHOOSE POLYUNSATURATED OR MONOUNSATURATED FATS IN PREFERENCE TO SATURATED ONES.

Vitamins and minerals

There are many vitamins and minerals and they are all vital for good health. If you are eating the right balance of carbohydrate, protein, and fat, then sufficient amounts of vitamins and minerals should be automatically included in the diet and supplements will not be necessary.

HEALTHY EATING – PUTTING IT INTO PRACTICE

More on carbohydrate

- All carbohydrate foods are eventually broken down into sugar. This group includes flour, bread, pasta, rice, potatoes, and breakfast cereals, as well as the sweet or sugar-containing foods which should be restricted.

- Remember, you should not cut out all the foods containing carbohydrate. This would merely encourage your body to produce more sugar from its reserves, which would cause you to lose weight and become unwell. Starvation is no treatment for any type of diabetes.

- You need to remember that your diet must contain enough carbohydrate to ensure a reasonable level of blood sugar, in order to produce the fuel your body needs for energy.

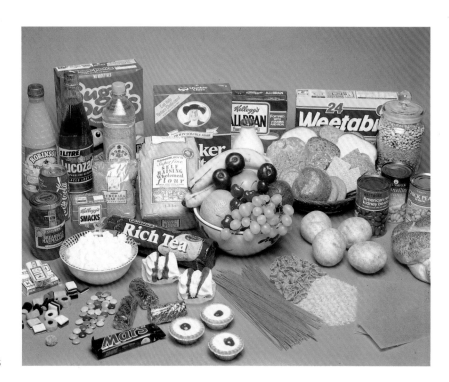

Fig. 3.7
Some common carbohydrate foods

The best choice of carbohydrate

Carbohydrate foods high in fibre, especially soluble fibre, help slow down the rise in blood sugar after a meal. This, of course, is much better for your diabetic control.

Carbohydrate foods high in fibre should make up about two-thirds of the carbohydrate you eat.

How to eat more fibre

● Eat wholemeal or granary bread rather than white. If you do not like either of these, then you could try high fibre white breads instead.

● Choose brown rice in preference to white. Remember, however, it takes about three times longer to cook and you will need about two to three times more water.

● Try experimenting with wholemeal flour. If you are used to baking with white flour, you may find the texture of wholemeal flour difficult to work with. Using half wholemeal and half white in recipes will give a lighter texture.

● At breakfast time, choose a wholewheat or oat based cereal. Avoid sugar coated ones.

● Make more use of beans, peas, and lentils. Add a few cooked beans to a casserole or stew to make the meat go further – this is cheaper and very nutritious. Remember to cook dried beans according the manufacturer's instructions.

● Fruit and vegetables are a very important part of the diet and provide fibre. Vegetables contain very small amounts of carbohydrate (sugar) and so, even if eaten in large amounts, should not affect your blood sugar level.

● Fruit is an excellent source of vitamins, but contains more sugar than vegetables. Enjoy fruit in your diet, but do not eat excessive amounts.

Fig. 3.8
Fruit and vegetables are essential for
a healthy diet

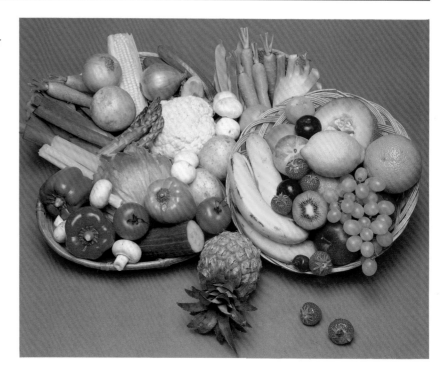

A word about carbohydrate exchanges

If you prefer to have more specific information about the amounts of food you should eat, your dietitian may advise you to eat specified amounts of carbohydrate foods at each meal.

One method of judging the amount of carbohydrate in each meal is by the **carbohydrate exchange system**. The dietitian will decide how much carbohydrate is needed each day, calculating this after looking at your weight, age, height, etc. The total amount of carbohydrate needed each day will be divided so that you eat most of it at main meals, with smaller amounts as snacks between meals.

Once you know how much carbohydrate to eat at each meal, you can then choose what you wish to eat using a carbohydrate exchange list.

Examples of foods containing 10 g of carbohydrate (or 1 'exchange') are shown in Fig. 3.9.

Fig. 3.9
A selection of exchanges

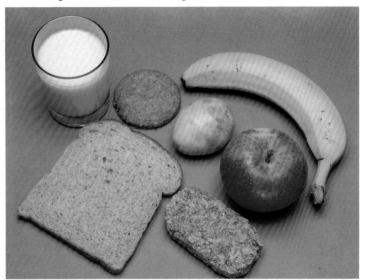

If it has been suggested, for example, that you need 50 g of carbohydrate or 5 exchanges at each meal you can simply select what you wish to eat from your exchange list. For 50 g of carbohydrate you could have two slices of bread, one Weetabix, one glass of milk, and one piece of fruit. Your snacks can be similarly varied. Your dietitian will be able to provide you with a more detailed list if necessary.

It is not necessary to weigh food. Carbohydrate exchanges can be calculated using simple household measures, such as a spoonful or a cupful. Remember, the amount of carbohydrate specified by your dietitian is only a general guide, not a rigid amount.

Do not be concerned if you have not come across this system. Most people with your type of diabetes do not usually need to follow a diet based on carbohydrate exchanges – it is more commonly used by people taking insulin treatment. Instead, those on diet and tablets, or on diet alone are advised to eat regularly, to eat an overall healthy balanced diet, and to have a source of carbohydrate at each meal.

Fig. 3.10
These foods are high in sugar and
should be restricted

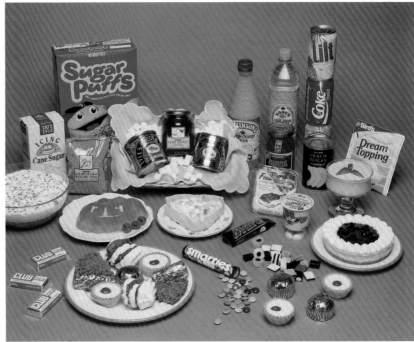

Foods to be restricted

Very sweet foods and drinks should be restricted in the diet, as they may cause a rapid rise in blood sugar. By restricting the amount of sweet foods you eat, you are minimizing the amount of sugar which has to be disposed of by your reduced insulin supply. A list of such foods is given in Table 1.

Table 1 Foods to be restricted
The foods listed below are high in sugar and have virtually no nutritional value
Marmalade*/jam*/honey
Mincemeat/lemon curd
Syrup and treacle/Sugar/Glucose/Glucose tablets
Fizzy and mixer drinks*, cordials*, and squashes*
Sweet pastries and cakes/Sweets and chocolates
Fruits tinned in syrup*
*Low sugar or sugar-free alternatives are available.

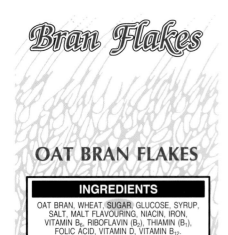

OAT BRAN FLAKES

INGREDIENTS

OAT BRAN, WHEAT, SUGAR, GLUCOSE, SYRUP, SALT, MALT FLAVOURING, NIACIN, IRON, VITAMIN B$_6$, RIBOFLAVIN (B$_2$), THIAMIN (B$_1$), FOLIC ACID, VITAMIN D, VITAMIN B$_{12}$.

Is sugar completely forbidden?

Many people feel that they must avoid sugar completely, and so check all food labels for traces of sugar. If you do this, you will soon find that many foods contain sugar, from tinned vegetables and baked beans to sauces, pickles, breakfast cereals, and bread. The amount of sugar present in such foods is small and is unlikely to affect your blood sugar levels. Therefore, we do not recommend that you avoid such foods. It is sweet, sugary foods which should be restricted. As a general guide, look at the label – the lower down the list of ingredients sugar appears, the less there is present in the product.

What can I use to sweeten food?

There is a wide range of artificial sweeteners available. All contain one or more of three sweeteners – aspartame, acesulfame K, or saccharin. All are virtually calorie and carbohydrate-free but, like any other additive, they should be taken only in moderation.

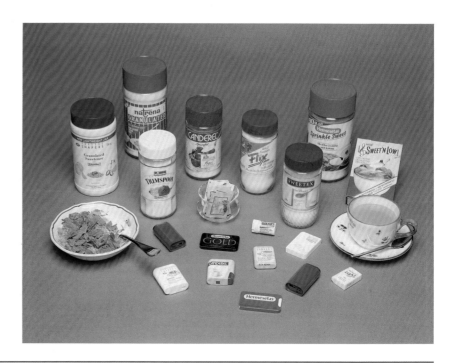

Fig. 3.11
Artificial sweeteners

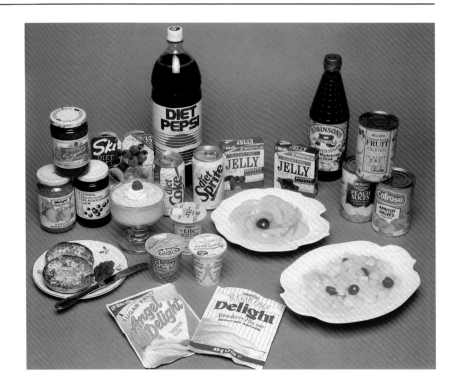

Fig. 3.12
There is a wide range of sugar-free
and reduced sugar products
available

Artificial sweeteners are readily available from most chemists and supermarkets, and are ideal for sweetening drinks, cereals, stewed fruits, and puddings. Most sweeteners are available in powder, liquid, or tablet form.

It is worth noting that aspartame-based sweeteners are destroyed by cooking, and so should be added just before serving. Sweeteners are not suitable for recipes where bulk is required, e.g. you would be unable to make a sponge cake using tablet sweeteners. Therefore, where artificial sweeteners cannot be used, it is suggested that small amounts of ordinary sugar (sucrose), up to 25 g (1 oz) per person per day, could be used in baking. Providing that the small amount of sugar is taken as part of an overall high fibre diet, it should not have a detrimental effect on your blood sugar.

Diabetic foods

Diabetic foods are not a necessary part of the diet. They are expensive and are often no lower in calories than their ordinary counterparts. For example, a bar of diabetic chocolate may have the same amount of fat and calories as a bar of ordinary chocolate.

Getting your fat intake right

Fat and fatty foods are high in calories and should be eaten in moderation. Therefore, cut down on the amount of fat and fatty foods you eat. This not only helps control your weight and your diabetes, but is also helpful in reducing the risk of arterial disease.

The fat in our food is a very concentrated source of calories – it can make up over half of the calories we eat, but should be limited to a third or less.

Most of the fat consumed comes from

- Fatty meat and meat products, e.g. beefburgers, sausages, meat pies
- Prepared manufactured foods, e.g. pastries, cakes, and biscuits
- Milk and dairy products, e.g. cheese, full fat milk, and cream
- Spreads and cooking fats, e.g. margarine, butter, lard and ghee.

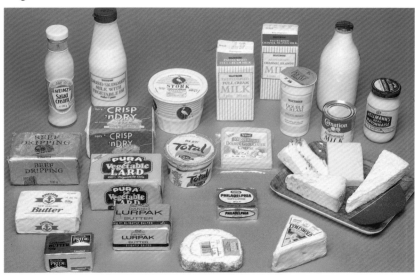

Fig. 3.13
Dairy products tend to be high in fat (lower fat versions are usually available)

Fig. 3.14
Fat is also 'hidden' in many foods

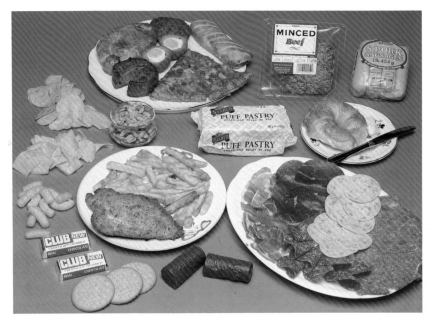

By following a few simple rules, it is possible to reduce your fat intake.

● Remove visible fat and skin from meat and poultry.

● Choose lean cuts of meat and try to include more fish and poultry in your diet.

● Try to avoid the frying pan – prepare by other cooking methods instead, e.g. baking, grilling or boiling.

● Cut down on the amount of high fat dairy products you eat, such as butter, cream, full fat cheese, and full fat milk. There are many low fat varieties available on the market, e.g. skimmed or semi-skimmed milk, low fat spreads, reduced fat creams and cheeses.

● Limit the amount of cakes, biscuits, and pastries you eat.

● Cut down on high fat snack foods, such as crisps and nuts.

● Most yogurts are low fat. Look for low fat, sugar-free varieties.

There is a wide range of reduced fat and fat-free products on the market (see Fig. 3.15).

Fig. 3.15
Reduced fat and fat free products

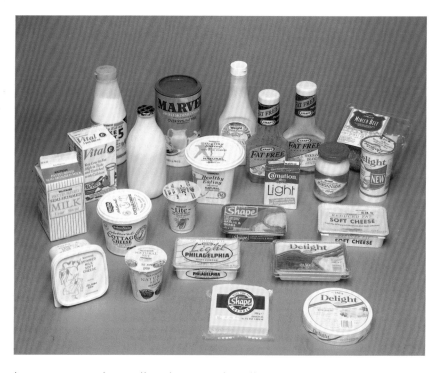

Go easy on salt

In some people, eating too much salt may lead to raised blood pressure. Therefore, try to cut down on the amount of salt you use by
- Eating fewer salty goods, such as processed meats, cheese and crisps
- Adding less salt to food during cooking
- Cutting down on the amount of salt added to food at the table.

Foods which can be eaten in generous quantities

Some foods are low in fat, sugar, and calories. They can be eaten in generous quantities. Examples are listed in Table 2.

Table 2 Foods which can be eaten freely

All vegetables, including

Cauliflower	Marrow	Tomatoes
Runner beans	Mushrooms	Peppers
Carrots	Celery	Swede
Onions	Turnips	Peas
Salad vegetables	Green leafy vegetables	

Fruit

Cranberries	Lemons	Rhubarb
Gooseberries	Loganberries	Redcurrants
Grapefruit		

Beverages

Tea	Bovril	Tomato juice
Coffee	Marmite	Lemon juice
Sugar-free squashes	Mixers	Soda water
Clear soups		

Seasonings

Pepper	Pickles	Spices
Mustard	Herbs	Stock cubes
Vinegar	Food colourings	Essences

Alcohol – what's your limit?

Having diabetes does not mean that you cannot drink alcohol, but it does mean that you must think more carefully about what you drink and when.

All types of alcoholic drinks contain calories. If you are overweight it is best not to have more than the occasional drink, and to count the calories into your daily allowance.

If you are taking chlorpropamide tablets for your diabetes, you may experience a hot flushing of the face after drinking alcohol. This is not dangerous, but can be very annoying. If this happens, discuss the matter with your doctor, who may be able to change the tablets. Some chemists put a 'do not drink alcohol' label on all prescriptions of diabetic tablets, but you may still be able to drink alcohol safely; ask your doctor.

Do not substitute alcoholic drinks for your usual meals, and never drink on an empty stomach. Although many alcoholic drinks contain small amounts of sugar, if the recommended alcohol allowance is not exceeded, the sugar content of the drink should not be enough to disturb your control.

Avoid the low sugar 'diet' lagers and beers. These tend to have a high alcohol content. Drink the ordinary varieties instead, preferably those with an alcohol content below 5 per cent.

Fig. 3.16
Drink alcohol in moderation

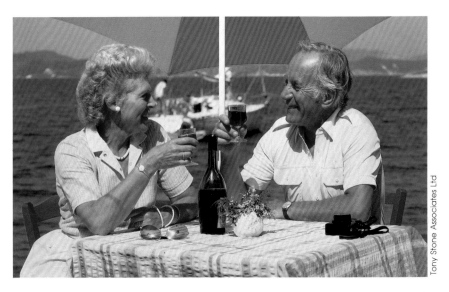

Alcohol-free and low alcohol beers, lagers, and wines are useful, especially if you are driving. However, they may be high in sugar and should be treated as a sugary drink. If drunk in moderation, they should not produce a rapid rise in your blood sugar level. If you are driving, check that your drink is an alcohol-free beverage, rather than just a reduced alcohol, one. It is possible to go over the limit if you drink too many low alcohol, as opposed to alcohol-free, drinks.

Always use low calorie mixers with spirits and be careful with home measures! Diluting your drink with plenty of low calorie mixer will make it last longer.

If you are out for the evening, it is a good idea to alternate alcoholic drinks with non-alcoholic ones. Soda water or low calorie tonic with ice and lemon can look like a sophisticated drink.

Excess alcohol is harmful for everybody, whether or not they have diabetes. Even if your weight is normal and blood sugar control good, it is recommended that men restrict alcohol intake to three units per day and women to two units per day. It is also suggested that you have two or three alcohol-free days each week.

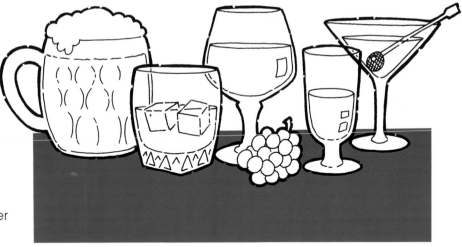

Fig. 3.17
1 unit of alcohol = $\frac{1}{2}$-pint lager, beer or cider, 1 glass of wine or sherry, liquer or aperitif

Remember
- **Never drink on an empty stomach**
- **Drink only in moderation**
- **Never drink and drive**
- **Always wear some form of diabetic identification.**

Your family's diet

Eating out

Fig. 3.18
The diet recommended for diabetes
is a healthy one, so all the family
would benefit from following such
a diet

Although the type of diet outlined is designed for the specific needs of a person with diabetes, it is a particularly healthy diet in so far as it is based on a low sugar and low fat intake, together with an increase in the consumption of fruit, vegetables, and fibre-containing foods. Consequently, it is recommended that the whole family should be offered the benefits of meals based on this type of diet.

As your knowledge of diet increases, you will gain more confidence when eating out, and you will be able to select those foods which you consider to be the best choice.

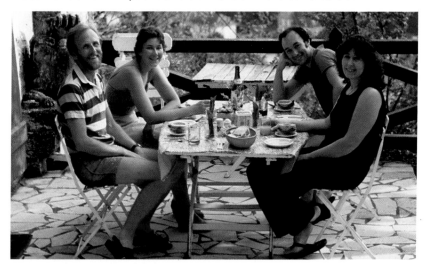

Eating with friends and relatives should pose no problems. If you let them know in advance which foods you prefer not to eat, any embarrassment will be easily avoided.

If you are at all concerned about the suitability of certain foods in a restaurant, do not be afraid to ask. Wherever possible

● Select generous portions of vegetables

● Avoid fatty and sugary foods

● Choose baked, grilled, or boiled foods, as opposed to fried or roasted.

However, an occasional indulgence, although it may lead to a temporary rise in blood sugar, will do no long-term harm.

If you are overweight

Most people (approximately 75 per cent) with your type of diabetes are overweight and it is therefore likely that you may be trying to correct this.

Weight loss is the most important measure needed to control blood sugar levels. It is very difficult to control your diabetes if you are overweight.

Some people can lose weight more quickly than others, but no one finds it easy. You have to look honestly at what you are actually eating and try to pinpoint areas where you could cut down. Are you eating lots of fatty foods, i.e. fatty meats, lots of butter, crisps, nuts, pastries, and pies? Are your portion sizes a bit on the large side? Are you eating late at night? Could you be making more use of low calorie or high fibre foods?

The type of diet you choose must be nutritionally balanced. Miracle diets and very low calorie diets can be tempting, but do not have long-term benefits.

Fig. 3.19
Are you overweight?

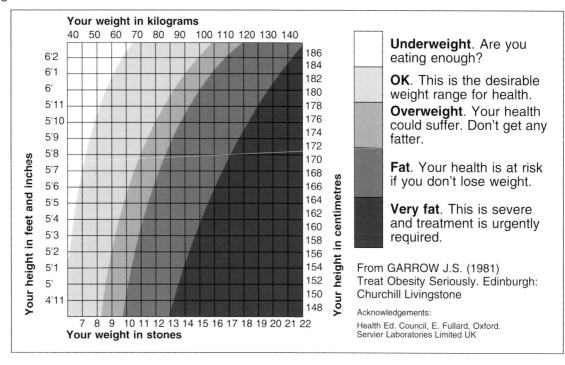

Your weight in kilograms

Your height in feet and inches

Your height in centimetres

Your weight in stones

Underweight. Are you eating enough?

OK. This is the desirable weight range for health.

Overweight. Your health could suffer. Don't get any fatter.

Fat. Your health is at risk if you don't lose weight.

Very fat. This is severe and treatment is urgently required.

From GARROW J.S. (1981) Treat Obesity Seriously. Edinburgh: Churchill Livingstone

Acknowledgements:

Health Ed. Council, E. Fullard, Oxford.
Servier Laboratories Limited UK

People vary in the way they wish to approach their weight reduction diet. Some prefer to follow general guidelines. They feel sufficiently in control not to have to plan meals strictly in advance and consider themselves capable of selecting the best choice at the time. Others are more comfortable if they plan in advance and determine exactly what each meal should contain.

Losing weight takes time – you put weight on slowly, and it takes a similar time to lose it again. Aim to lose $\frac{1}{2}$–1 kg (1–2 lb) each week. You may lose a little more at the start of your diet, but this is mainly water, not fat. Because your weight fluctuates, you should not be tempted to weigh yourself every day. Instead, weigh yourself once a week, preferably on the same day, and first thing in the morning.

You should set yourself a realistic target weight, which you should discuss with your dietitian. Aim for a moderate weight loss to start with, and once you have achieved this, set a new target if necessary.

Asking your family doctor to refer you to a State Registered Dietitian is the most sensible approach. A dietitian can recommend a calorie intake and eating plan which suits your lifestyle, is medically safe, and which contains the correct balance of nutrients.

Hints on dietary control

● **Never miss a meal** or you will be extremely hungry at the next one and may then find it difficult to stick to your diet. You will lose weight more easily if you eat more regular meals, rather than saving up your calories for a large supper at the end of the day.

● **You may find it useful to plan your meals the day before**. If you know what you are going to eat at each meal, then you will not be tempted to take the first thing you see in the cupboard.

● **Avoid diabetic products**. Most are high in calories and fat.

● **Always try to sit down to eat a meal** – it is surprising how much you can eat without noticing it when you are on the move!

● **Do not prepare too much food**. If there are two of you in the family, prepare meals for two, not four. You will be tempted by the left-overs, as no one likes to see food being thrown away.

● **Have plenty of low calorie foods (e.g. salads and vegetables) to hand for when hunger strikes.**

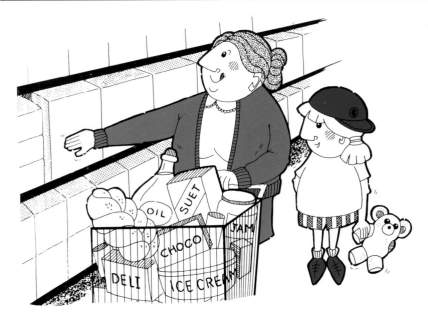

- **Never shop when you are hungry**, or you will be tempted to buy more. It may help to make a shopping list: if you keep to it, you will be less likely to need to go into the supermarket aisles where they keep the cakes and sweets.
- **If you have to buy sweets and crisps for your family, try to avoid bulk buying**. If you have children who are fond of chocolate, buy them just one bar at a time, rather than a packet containing several bars – having the extra bars around is simply putting temptation in your way. If possible, persuade your family to buy their own treats and to eat them when you are not around.

More about amounts of food

The following tables are provided to give you a guide to the changes you can make, depending on whether you need to lose or maintain your weight.

The first column shows examples of typical meals which you may have been eating before your diabetes was discovered.

The right hand column should be used by those not trying to lose weight. This column shows you the changes that you could make to your diet to enable you to have more fibre, less fat, and less sugar, without affecting the calorie content, and yet have similar types of food.

The column in the middle is for those trying to lose weight. It shows you the changes you could make to your diet to enable you to eat fewer calories and yet still have plenty of variety in your meals.

Table – 3 Breakfast

Typical meal	Changes to be made to help you lose weight	Changes to be made if you are normal weight
Sweetened fruit juice 1 bowl of sugar-coated cereal Full fat milk Sugar	Unsweetened fruit juice 1 small bowl of wholewheat cereal Skimmed or semi-skimmed milk Artificial sweetener, if desired	Unsweetened fruit juice 1 bowl of wholewheat cereal and sliced banana Skimmed or semi-skimmed milk Artificial sweetener, if desired
White toast Butter Jam	1–2 small slices of wholemeal or granary toast Scraping of polyunsaturated margarine or low fat spread Scraping of reduced sugar jam	Wholemeal or granary toast Scraping of polyunsaturated margarine or low fat spread Scraping of reduced sugar jam
Fried sausages Fried eggs Toasted white bread Butter Marmalade	Scrambled egg and tomato 1–2 small toasted slices of wholemeal or granary bread Scraping of polyunsaturated margarine or low fat spread Scraping of reduced sugar marmalade	Grilled sausages Scrambled egg and tomato Toased wholemeal or granary bread Scraping of polyunsaturated margarine or low fat spread Scraping of reduced sugar marmalade

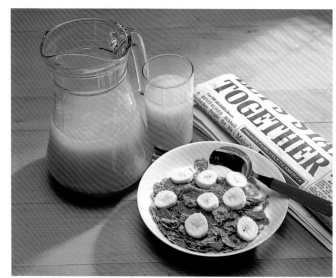

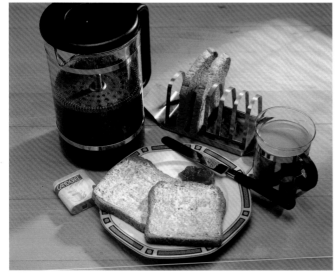

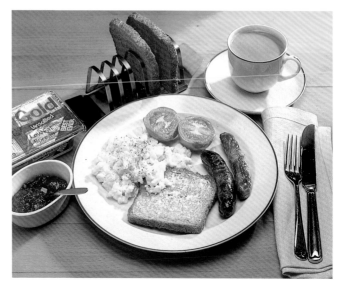

Table – 4 Light meals

Typical Meal	Changes to be made to help you lose weight	Changes to be made if you are normal weight
Jacket potato Butter Large portion of cheese Fruit yoghurt	Small jacket potato Polyunsaturated margarine or low fat spread Cottage cheese, sweetcorn Salad Sugar-free fruit yoghurt	Jacket potato Polyunsaturated margarine or low fat spread Small portion of cheese, sweetcorn Salad Sugar-free fruit yoghurt Piece of fruit
Egg mayonnaise sandwich made with white bread Crisps Fruit	Small egg salad sandwich made with wholemeal or granary bread Fruit	Egg salad sandwich made with wholemeal or granary bread Low fat crisps Fruit
Cheese hamburger (4 oz)	Grilled hamburger (2 oz) with wholemeal roll Salad	Grilled hamburger (4 oz) with large wholemeal roll Salad Fruit

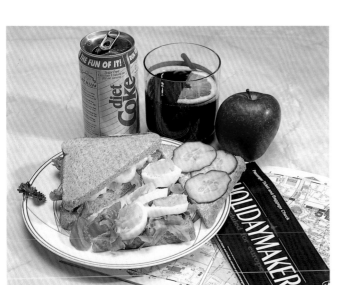

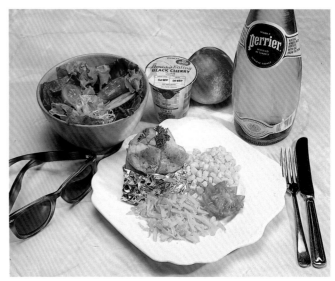

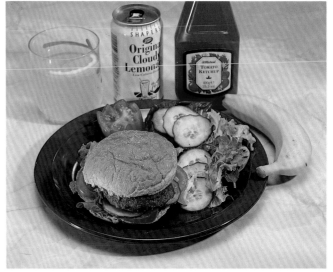

Table 5 – Main meals

Typical meal	Changes to be made to help you lose weight	Changes to be made if you are normal weight
Roast chicken (including skin) Roast potatoes, small portion of vegetables with butter Tinned fruit and ice-cream	Roast chicken (without skin) Small portion of jacket or boiled potatoes, large portion of vegetables – no butter Tinned fruit in natural juice	Roast chicken (without skin) Large jacket or boiled potatoes, large portion of vegetables – no butter Tinned fruit in natural juice and ice-cream
Fried fish in breadcrumbs Chips, peas Apple pie with custard	Grilled fish in breadcrumbs Small jacket potato, peas Fresh fruit salad and natural yogurt	Grilled fish in breadcrumbs Oven ready chips (reduced fat), peas Apple pie made with half wholemeal, half white flour, with artificial sweetener Custard made with skimmed milk with artificial sweetener
White spaghetti, bolognaise sauce, cheese on top Cheesecake	Small portion of wholewheat spaghetti, small portion of bolognaise sauce Side salad Diet yoghurt	Wholewheat spaghetti, bolognaise sauce Side salad Cheesecake made with artifical sweetener and low fat cheese

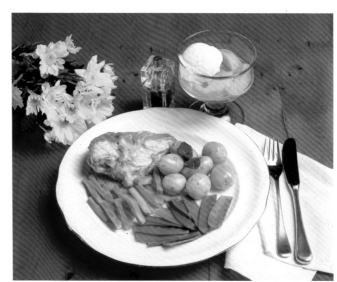

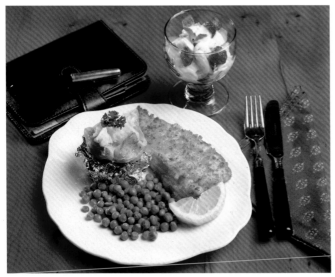

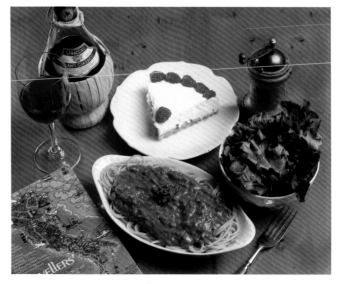

Summary

- Eat regular meals.
- If you are overweight try very hard to lose weight
  - set yourself a target to aim for
  - do not expect too much too soon
  - once you have lost weight don't let it creep up again.
- Watch your fat intake and avoid eating lots of fat and fatty foods.
- Control your sugar intake by restricting your intake of sweet and sugary foods.
- Eat plenty of high fibre foods, including fruit and vegetables.
- Use salt in moderation.
- Take care with alcohol.
- Try and take regular, frequent exercise.

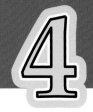

Tablet treatment

Sometimes treatment with diet alone is not entirely successful. In such circumstances tablets may need to be taken in combination with your diet. This chapter describes the tablets, how and when you should take them, and answers questions you may have about side effects and alteration of the dose.

Which tablets to use

Two types of tablets are usually used to treat non-insulin dependent diabetes. The tablets that work by stimulating your pancreas to produce more insulin are the more common. These are listed in Table 6.

Occasionally, however, these tablets are not completely effective if used alone. In such cases an additional tablet, called metformin (trade name Glucophage) may also be prescribed. Metformin may sometimes be used on its own, especially if you are overweight.

Remember, too, that you must stick to your diet when taking tablets. You cannot expect the tablets to control your sugar level if you eat what you like – they are not a substitute for diet!

Table 6 – Tablets used to treat diabetes

Chemical name	Brand name
SULPHONYLUREA TYPE	
Acetohexamide	Dimelor
Chlorpropamide	Diabinese, Glymese, Melitase
Glibenclamide	Daonil, Semi-daonil, Euglucon, Libanil, Malix
Glibornuride	Glutril
Gliclazide	Diamicron
Glipizide	Glibenese, Minodiab
Gliquidone	Glurenorm
Glymidine	Gondafon
Tolazamide	Tolanase
Tolbutamide	Glyconon, Pramidex, Rastinon
BIGUANIDE TYPE	
Metformin	Glucophage

Some important questions about tablet treatment

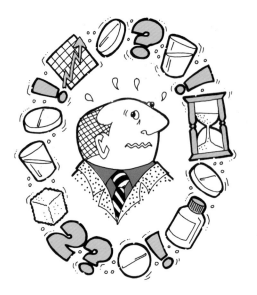

When should tablets be taken?

Usually, they are prescribed to be taken either once a day first thing in the morning before breakfast, or twice a day before breakfast and before your evening meal.

Can I relax my diet?

No. Unfortunately tablets will only work **in addition** to your diet. If you relax your diet, good control is most unlikely.

Am I at risk until my blood sugar returns to normal?

Initially, your treatment with diet, or with a combination of diet and tablets, will take a few weeks to return your blood sugar to a normal level. During this period, however, you will come to no harm. The long-term complications of diabetes, which affect the eyes, kidneys, and nerves, take many years to develop.

What happens if the tablets do not work?

If your blood sugar remains high, in spite of taking tablets, and you are carefully following your diet, your doctor may recommend insulin. In the majority of people, however, this is never necessary. Most instances of difficulty with control are due to a failure to follow the diet.

Is there a risk of going into a diabetic coma?

No, this is very rare in your type of diabetes. Diabetic coma occurs when there is a complete absence of insulin. Fat breakdown products build up in the blood, a process which takes place over several hours and can eventually lead to coma. It never happens when you are well. If you should become sick, vomit, lose your appetite and become very thirsty, and your tests (see Chapter 5) are positive, you should consult your doctor to be on the safe side.

Can the blood sugar go too low?

Yes. This is called hypoglycaemia and can occur with tablet treatment (but not with diet alone), although only rarely. It is usually easily recognized, as you will feel sweaty, hungry, and possibly faint. In particular, it may occur if you have not eaten for some time.

Table 7 – Recognizing hypoglycaemia

The common symptoms of hypoglycaemia include

- Trembling
- Sweating
- Tingling around the mouth
- Palpitations of the heart, and then
  - Difficulty in concentration
  - Confusion
  - Muzziness
  - Faintness
  - Headache
  - Blurring of vision
  - Unsteadiness
  - Irritability, bad temper
  - Unusual lack of co-operation.

If my blood sugar goes too low, what should I do?

Immediately have something to eat or drink that contains sugar, e.g. two digestive biscuits, a Mars bar, or some sweetened fruit juice. If the symptoms do not disappear within a few minutes, have something more to eat. Sometimes, the feelings come back an hour or so later. If this happens, you should have some more to eat. If the symptoms recur on more than one day, or if they do not disappear after you have eaten something, then you will need to see your doctor. You should tell your doctor, anyway, on your next visit. The dosage of the tablets may need adjusting.

Can tablets cause other side effects?

Side effects are rare. The sulphonylurea tablets cause no serious ill effects in the many thousands of people who take them. Slight swelling of the ankles may be noted in the early stages of treatment, and weight gain of a few pounds can occur. Skin rashes occur very occasionally.

Diarrhoea or abdominal pains are not uncommon at the start of treatment with metformin but usually wear off. If they persist, stop the metformin tablets and consult your doctor.

If you are taking chlorpropamide tablets you may develop flushing of the face after drinking alcohol. Although discomforting, it is quite harmless and lasts only a few minutes. There is no need to stop drinking alcohol but, if the problem becomes troublesome, a change of tablet might be considered.

Can I drive with tablet treatment?

Yes (but see section on Driving, page 84). If you do have any odd feelings that might be due to hypoglycaemia be very careful. The symptoms (described in Table 7) may interfere with concentration and ability to drive. Stop immediately and have something to eat. You should always carry some biscuits or something similar in the car, just in case. Do not start to drive again until you feel better. Do not drive at all if you feel unwell.

Are there any other alternative treatments?

A number of remedies have been tried. These include tablets, called 'starch splitters', to reduce the absorption of carbohydrates from food. They appear to have very limited success and may cause diarrhoea. Attempts have also been made to delay the absorption of starch using guar. Unfortunately, the dose may need to be very high to be effective, and therefore it is often unpleasant to take.

Summary

- Tablet treatment is used when changes in the diet provide insufficient control.
- Tablets have very few side effects and in most people none at all.
- Metformin tablets can cause stomach disturbance, but this can usually be avoided by starting on a low dose.
- Occasionally, low blood sugars can occur – if you suspect this, have something to eat straight away.

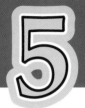

Is your treatment effective?

The aim of diabetes treatment is to return and keep your blood sugar within normal limits.

Unfortunately, **how you feel is not a reliable guide to the level of your blood sugar**. Symptoms, such as thirst, weight loss, and passing large amounts of urine, appear **only if the diabetes is badly out of control**. Even with moderately high levels of blood sugar – the sort of levels which can, over a period of years, lead to serious complications – you may have no symptoms. Therefore, it is important to ensure that your diabetic control is being maintained at an acceptable level. This chapter describes simple tests which enable you to check that your treatment is effective.

Blood tests v. urine tests

Blood sugar levels can be assessed either directly by means of blood tests, or indirectly by urine tests. Urine tests have the important advantage that they are painless. Also, because they are much simpler to perform, they can easily be carried out at home. Therefore, for many of those with non-insulin dependent diabetes, regular urine testing will provide an effective guide to blood sugar levels.

Blood tests will be carried out when you attend the clinic or visit your doctor, in order to check that your urine tests are providing reliable information about your actual blood picture.

For some people, urine tests can be misleading, because they fail to record high levels when they should. If the tests performed when you attend your clinic or doctor reveal this, you will be advised to perform blood tests.

Some may feel unhappy about handling urine, although in most people it is perfectly sterile and clean. The techniques now available for self blood sugar testing make it possible for you to avoid urine tests, if you so wish. An increasing number of people prefer to use the blood testing method.

Blood tests require only a single drop of blood, which you can obtain by pricking your finger. The test only takes a couple of minutes to do, but must be carried out carefully to ensure an accurate result. Most people with non-insulin dependent diabetes do not need to perform direct measurements of their blood sugar routinely.

Urine tests

How urine tests work and their interpretation

When the blood sugar rises, a point is reached at which it starts to leak into the urine. In the majority of people this will happen whenever the blood sugar is too high, usually above about 10 mmol/l. Therefore, if the blood sugar has exceeded this threshold level since you last passed urine, a test for sugar in the urine will be **positive** (Fig. 5.1a). If the blood sugar is below this level (normal), the urine tests will be **negative** (Fig. 5.1b).

Fig. 5.1
How urine tests work

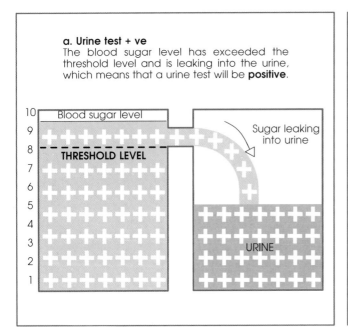
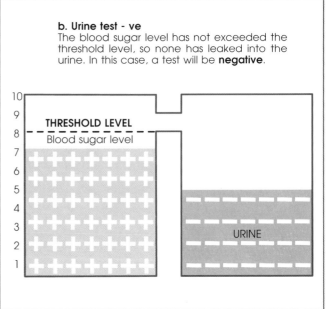

What should you aim for?

Your doctor should discuss with you the level of diabetes control for which you should aim. You should ask for this information, as it is very difficult to achieve something if you do not know what you are aiming for. To assess the control of diabetes the sugar levels in the body are tested.

Normally, the blood sugar should not rise above a certain level (9–10 mmol/l), as shown in Fig. 5.1a. When the blood sugar rises above about 8 mmol/l in most people, sugar spills into the urine. Therefore, when you test your urine, it should be free of sugar. You will be encouraged to keep your blood tests below 10 mmol/l and your urine free of sugar.

What should you do if the tests are high?

An occasional reading out of the normal range is acceptable. Sometimes a high or low reading is unexplainable. Usually high readings can be related to extra stress, less exercise, eating more than normal, or perhaps forgetting your diabetes tablets. Low readings may be linked to taking more exercise than usual, or forgetting or delaying a meal.

Another time when you might expect to get high readings is if you are feeling ill. Illness increases the blood sugar levels and, as with high urine tests, repeated high blood tests may indicate the need for a temporary change in treatment.

How often should you do tests?

To start with you will be asked to test several times a day, because this will help you to understand what causes the blood sugar to rise. As your urine tests become negative, i.e. as your blood sugar returns to normal, two or three tests a week may be sufficient to reassure you that all remains well. Stress and illness also increase your blood sugar. Therefore, you would be wise to test your urine several times a day during any illness – even a cold or flu – in order to discover whether your treatment is still effective.

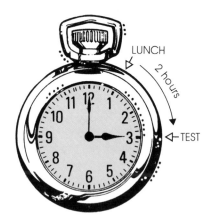

LUNCH
2 hours
TEST

When should you test?

Once treatment has begun to take effect, you will only wish to know if at any time the blood sugar is abnormally high. Therefore, you should perform your urine test two hours after a main meal, since it is at this time that your blood sugar will be at its highest. If you feel unwell, it is wise to test first thing in the morning, before breakfast, and before other meals as well.

Keep a record of your tests

Isolated tests of the urine are of little value, but a regular record (Fig. 5.2) gives a much better idea of the level of control being achieved. Such a record will be of particular value when you attend your doctor or clinic for your regular medical check-up. Each test should be recorded on a chart or in a book.

Fig. 5.2
Keep a record of your urine tests

Date / Time	Urine Glucose				Remarks:
	8am	2.30 pm	6pm	10pm	
Mon	nil				
Tue	nil				
Wed		++			After meal
Thur	nil				
Fri				nil	
Sat					
Sun	+++				Heavy meal night before

How are urine tests performed?

There are various urine tests available and they are all quite satisfactory. The main brands are Diastix and Diabur-Test 5000 (test strips). All the tests involve placing test strips in urine and observing a colour change. You will, of course, be shown how to test your urine when you first develop diabetes. If you have any doubts as to whether you are doing it correctly, check with your doctor or clinic. Urine tests depend on a colour change, so if you cannot see well, or if you are colour blind, you may not be able to detect the change and the tests may need to be done for you.

Fig. 5.3
Urine test kits
Diastix ▽   Diabur-Test 5000 ▷

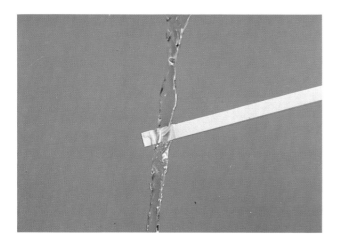

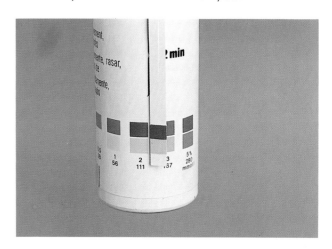

Blood tests

Blood testing technique

Blood tests should be performed carefully. It is easy to get an inaccurate result if the correct technique is not followed. The doctor or nurse should instruct you in the proper procedure and how to read the results of your blood tests. Most people read the results by matching the change in colour of the strip against a colour chart on the strip container. Alternatively, it is possible to purchase a blood glucose meter (they are not available on prescription) which will measure the colour change. Although a meter gives you a more precise reading, it does not make the test any more accurate. You still need to carry out the technique carefully.

If you can 'read' the strip by comparing it with the chart, there is **no need** to purchase a meter. Some meters use strips which cannot be read by eye. If you do decide to purchase a meter there are many to choose from, and you will find them advertised in the BDA's magazine *Balance*.

As with urine tests, blood tests are best performed 1–2 hours after a meal or, if you are unwell, before each meal. It is worth writing the results down, so that you can discuss their meaning with your doctor.

Fig. 5.4
Record the results of your blood tests

| MONTH APRIL | | TEST TIME | | | | | | | COMMENTS |
Day	Date	Before B/Fast	After B/Fast	Before Lunch	After Lunch	Before Dinner	Evening	Before Bed	MEDICATION, ILLNESS, ETC.
MON	1	6.0							Diabetes tablet 2 daily
TUES	2		11.0						
WED	3								
THURS	4				12.0				
FRID	5								
SAT	6						7.0		
SUN	7	4.0							
	8								
	9								
	10								
	11								
	12								
	13								
	14								
	15								
	16								

Availability of testing strips

Most testing materials for urine or blood are available on prescription. Meters for reading strips have to be purchased (approximately £25–60).

High readings

If you are getting frequent high readings (greater than 8.0 mmol/l) you need to ask your doctor if your treatment needs modifying in some way.

Long-term tests

Blood tests which measure control over a period of time are the glycosylated haemoglobin test and the fructosamine test. These blood tests show the average blood sugars over the last two to six weeks. One of these tests should be performed when you attend the clinic or family doctor. You should ask about the results of these tests when you see your doctor.

Regular weighing

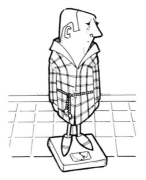

You will be advised of the most appropriate weight for your height, and be given a target to aim for if you are overweight. If your weight is normal, occasional weight checks are also important as an increase may well cause a deterioration in your diabetic control.

Unexpected loss of weight may indicate all is not going well, and if this happens do discuss it with your doctor.

When diabetes goes out of control

Factors leading to loss of control

In certain circumstances diabetes may go out of control unexpectedly. These are the five most common causes of loss of control.

1. **The development of an acute infection**
   - Urinary infection
   - Large boils, carbuncles, or abscesses
   - Severe chest infection
   - More seriously – gastroenteritis associated with vomiting.

2. **After starting certain medications**
   - Especially with steroids (prednisone, cortisone)
   - Sometimes with certain water tablets (diuretics) used in the treatment of high blood pressure and heart disease.

3. **Stressful situations**
   When people with diabetes are worried or anxious, they may find that their diabetes becomes more difficult to control.

4. **Failure to respond to tablets**
   In some people with diabetes, the tablets may lose their effect after a period of satisfactory control. Changing to a different tablet may correct the situation, but a few people may need to be re-stabilized with insulin.

5. **Failure to follow the advised treatment**
   People with diabetes who abandon their diet, stop taking their tablets, or both, will almost certainly become badly controlled, although the deterioration may be quite a gradual process.

What you need to do

In any of these situations, the blood sugar may rise and large amounts of sugar may be passed in the urine. Most illnesses, such as flu and colds, are of short duration and have no significant long-term effects, though the blood sugar, and hence urine tests, may show increases for a day or so. An occasional dietary indiscretion may also show itself in a similar way. If, however, the urine test becomes positive for sugar for more than a couple of days, **you may need additional treatment and you should contact your doctor**.

Vomiting and severe diarrhoea are, however, of greater significance, because they may cause the loss of a substantial amount of fluid and consequently an increased thirst. Although a person with non-insulin dependent diabetes does not develop ketoacidosis (diabetic coma), the salt balance in the blood may become disturbed.

You must consult your family doctor

● If you have had plenty of fluid to drink, but you still feel thirsty and unwell, and

● All your urine tests are positive, or

● Your blood tests are more than 15 mmol/l.

Very rarely, your doctor may decide you need admission to hospital, so that the large quantity of fluid you have lost can be replaced by intravenous drip, and also because insulin may be required, at least temporarily.

Summary

● Some regular checks are essential to see if your treatment is working.
● You should perform these checks at least twice a week and more often if you are having problems.
● Urine tests are usually quite satisfactory for the majority of people with your type of diabetes.
● Some may prefer blood testing, which is quite easy to perform.
● Blood tests are essential for some people, because their urine tests can give misleading information.
● It is wise to have a long-term blood test (HbA1) from time to time to check that your own tests are accurate.

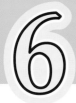

Insulin treatment

Sometimes, despite sticking to your diet and additional treatment with tablets, your sugar levels may continue to be too high. If this happens it is possible your doctor will recommend insulin treatment. Although there is quite a lot to learn when starting insulin injections, this chapter summarizes what you can expect. More detailed information is provided in the book *Insulin Dependent Diabetes*, which is also published by the British Diabetic Association.

It must be remembered that any treatment takes several weeks or sometimes months to work. Fortunately, insulin treatment for people with your type of diabetes is rather easier than for people with insulin dependent diabetes who are producing no insulin at all. Although you are still producing insulin, the amount may be insufficient to prevent the blood sugar from remaining at too high a level. The decision to start insulin will usually only be taken when your doctor is sure the tablet treatment has not worked.

Important aspects of insulin treatment

Why injections?

Unfortunately, if insulin is taken by mouth it is simply digested and destroyed before it gets properly into the body. For this reason it has to be given by injection. You will therefore have to learn to give the injections yourself. This, however, is much easier than you might think: the syringe is small and the needle very fine. Most people find that it hurts very little.

Overall aims of insulin treatment

The main purpose of treatment with injections is to copy the normal situation, i.e. to provide levels of insulin in the blood similar to those found in people whose insulin production is working normally. Figure 2.4 on page 13 shows how insulin is normally released into the blood after meals. The level rises as the sugar level rises, and falls again as the effect of the meal wears off. The blood sugar returns to normal under the influence of the insulin.

Fig. 6.1
Injecting insulin is much easier and
less painful than you might think

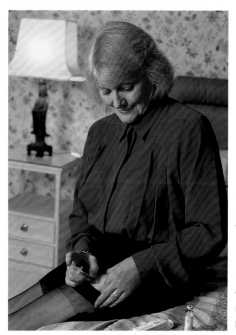

The aim, therefore, is to provide a peak of insulin at the times when the blood sugar is highest. Since it takes a little while for the insulin to get from the injection site into the circulation, this means giving it 30 minutes or so before a meal. The injections usually have to be given twice a day. Some people find it easier to have smaller, more frequent injections with a larger injection at night. The intention will be to find the right combination of number and timing of injections to return your blood sugar to normal throughout the day.

What happens if you have too much insulin?

The blood sugar will fall too low if too large a dose of insulin is given. This is a condition known as hypoglycaemia or, for short, a 'hypo'. It is also sometimes referred to as an 'insulin reaction', or just a 'reaction'. When this happens a number of symptoms occur. These include sweating, fainting, hunger, or palpitations. You will be taught to recognize the symptoms and you should take sugar or a sugary drink **as soon** as you feel them coming on. It usually only takes a few minutes before you feel normal again. Very rarely, if the symptoms are not recognized, you may become unconscious. Eventually you will come round, as the body restores the sugar level to normal and the insulin effect wears off. No harm should come to you, but prevention is better than cure. If you do not miss meals and snacks and you check your blood sugar regularly, especially during the early stages of your treatment, you should be able to avoid hypos fairly easily. Fortunately, these reactions are very uncommon in your type of diabetes.

Testing

Up until now you may have only used urine testing. This, however, will only tell you how high the sugar has been. Urine tests give you no indication of the low blood sugars which might lead to hypoglycaemia. With insulin treatment the blood sugar changes more quickly and to a greater extent than with diet or tablets. In the first instance you will need to test to find out the correct doses and frequency of injections, and the right balance between injections and meals. You will want to make adjustments in order to fit your insulin treatment into your daily life without too many changes. For this reason it is recommended that blood testing is performed, which will give you a much more accurate picture of what is going on. Further details of urine and blood tests are given in Chapter 5.

Is insulin treatment for ever?

Usually, yes. Once it has been decided that you are not producing enough insulin to remain well, the insulin injections will probably need to be continued permanently. Sometimes, however, insulin treatment may be used as a temporary measure when some other illness makes your diabetes more difficult to control than usual. For example, this might happen after a heart attack, an operation, or a serious infection. The insulin will then be stopped as you recover.

During pregnancy, insulin may be started to ensure perfect control while you are carrying the baby. It will be discontinued when your baby is born.

Does the dose keep on going up?

No. Once you have worked out your usual daily dose, this will not change to any major degree. However, your blood sugar may vary according to what you do or eat. Day-by-day variation is common. You may therefore have to make small adjustments on a day-to-day basis to fit in with your lifestyle. You may need an increased dose if you develop another illness, but these increases are usually temporary.

Does the diet need adjusting?

You cannot relax your diet completely once you have started insulin. If you do, your weight will increase and the insulin will work less efficiently. Therefore, you will have to continue to watch your total calorie intake. Sugar and sweet sugary foods are still not advisable as they will produce very rapid increases of blood sugar. These are difficult to correct without large and frequent doses of insulin, which will increase the risk of hypoglycaemia. One thing that is necessary, is to ensure that your meals are taken regularly. If you miss meals after taking your insulin, the risk of too low a blood sugar (hypoglycaemia) is high. It may also be advisable to have small snacks last thing at night.

You should be able to undertake normal sporting activities, work (including working shifts), and physical exercise, etc. You may, however, have to make some adjustments in the carbohydrate you eat and in your insulin doses. Most people quickly learn how to do this, with the help of the clinic if necessary.

Driving

Particular care is needed while driving. This is to prevent hypoglycaemia, which could cause an accident.

- Always test yourself before a journey.
- Don't drive for too long without a meal or snack.
- Always carry sugar with you in case you get any of the symptoms of hypoglycaemia.
- Always stop if you do get any such symptoms.
- Inform the DVLC and your insurance company that you have started insulin injections (see page 84).

Insulin injections and normal daily activities

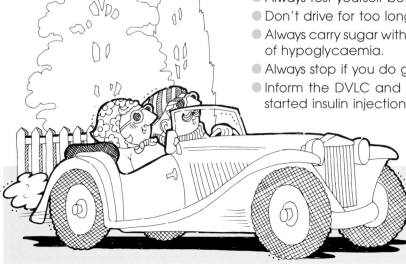

How will taking insulin affect my work?

Most people are able to continue with their normal work. Unfortunately, certain jobs are forbidden to those taking insulin, including joining the armed services, the police, or the fire service. Exceptions may be made, however, for serving members who have to start injections after treatment with diet and tablets. Driving public service vehicles, trains, or heavy goods vehicles, and flying aircraft are normally not allowed. For most jobs, therefore, there should be no problems. If, however, you do a job in which temporary loss of consciousness might cause you or others to be in danger, then you need to discuss this with your doctor.

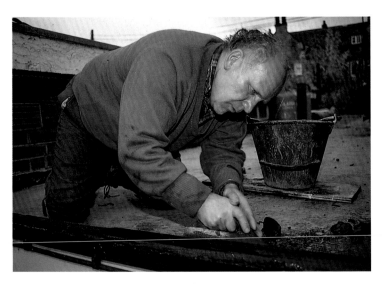

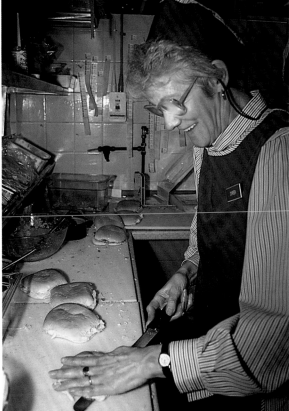

Fig. 6.2
Most People with diabetes can continue with their normal work

More information

If you do have to start insulin treatment you will require more information. This is provided in the book *Insulin Dependent Diabetes*, which is also published by the BDA.

Summary

- Insulin treatment may be necessary for some people with your type of diabetes.
- This will only be necessary if diet, or diet and tablet treatment is unsuccessful.
- Insulin is easier to give than most people expect, but does have to be given by injection.
- Full instructions will be provided to make this as easy for you as possible.

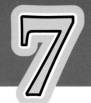
This chapter describes the possible long-term effects of diabetes, how they may affect you, and the sort of treatment that can be given. An outline is also provided of the type of medical care and supervision you should expect.

Treatment of diabetes very rapidly restores health to normal. The symptoms disappear quite quickly and any loss of weight or of energy soon return to normal.

After many years of diabetes, however, some of the body's tissues may be damaged. The eyes, kidneys, and some nerves (mainly those to the feet) are most susceptible. These problems are likely to develop **only** after many years of poor blood sugar control. Therefore, they are preventable by the majority of people. Many are completely spared these problems and, even after more than 40 years of diabetes, show no trace of any complications.

Damage to the feet

Foot problems are rather common in your type of diabetes, but can usually be prevented with care. Therefore, this section is particularly important to you.

Long-term diabetes sometimes results in nerve damage (called neuritis or neuropathy). This mainly affects the feeling in the feet.

The feet normally undergo a lot of wear and tear, and any injuries are usually noticed because of discomfort. If, however, discomfort is not felt because of neuritis, increasing damage to the feet may pass unnoticed. In addition, these injuries may be further aggravated by diminished circulation, which may lead to ulceration and infection. This can be very serious and result in prolonged periods off work, in bed, or in hospital, and sometimes requires operations or even amputations.

To a large extent these injuries can be avoided, if proper care is taken of the feet.

The 'do's' and 'don'ts' of foot care are of great importance, and you should read the following section carefully.

Prevention of foot problems

Scrupulous attention to care of the feet can prevent serious complications.

General measures for everyone

- Try and keep as good control of your diabetes as possible. This will keep the risk of any problems to a minimum.
- Avoid smoking. Nicotine is particularly harmful to the circulation of the lower legs and feet. The risk of severe changes is greatly increased if you continue to smoke.
- Be careful with your choice of footwear. Avoid shoes that rub, causing hard skin (callus) or blistering. Excess moisture may be a problem with sports shoes and lead to fungal infections.
- Wash your feet regularly and ensure that they are dried properly, especially between the toes.
- Learn how to cut your nails correctly.

Nail cutting

- When your toenails need cutting, do it after bathing, when the nails are soft and pliable. Do not cut them too short.
- Never cut the corners of your nails too far back at the sides, but allow the cut to follow the natural line of the end of the toe.
- Never use a sharp instrument to clean under your nails or in the nail grooves at the sides of the nails.
- If your toe nails are painful, or if you experience difficulty in cutting them, consult a State Registered Chiropodist.

Regular examination

- Make sure your feet are examined every year. This is the only way to find out whether greater care is necessary.

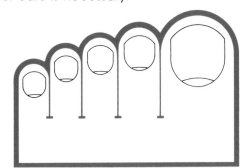

Special measures for older people

For older people and those in whom signs of nerve or blood vessel damage have been detected, the following measures and precautions are ESSENTIAL.

Inspecting your feet

- Inspect your feet regularly – ideally, daily – and if you cannot do this yourself, ask a friend to do it for you. This inspection is important, because you may not always be able to feel bruises or sores.
- Seek advice if you develop any cracks or breaks in the skin, any calluses or corns, or your feet are swollen or throbbing. Free advice from a State Registered Chiropodist should be available under the National Health Service.

Washing your feet

- Wash your feet daily in warm water, but do not soak them.
- Use a mild type of toilet soap.
- Rinse the skin well after washing. Dry your feet carefully, blotting between the toes with a soft towel.
- Dust with unperfumed talcum powder, wiping off any excess and ensuring that it does not clog between the toes.

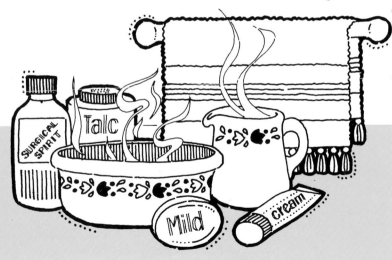

- If your skin is too dry, sparingly apply a little moisturising cream or an emulsifying ointment. This should be gently rubbed in after bathing the feet.
- If your skin is too moist, wipe your feet with surgical spirit, especially between the toes. When the spirit has dried, dust the skin with talcum powder.

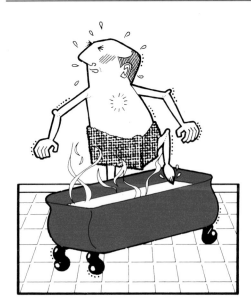

Heat and cold

- Be careful to avoid baths that are too hot.
- Do not sit too close to heaters or fires, and protect your legs and feet by covering them with a rug.
- Before getting into bed, remove hot-water bottles, unless they are fabric covered. Electric under-blankets should be switched off and unplugged.
- Do not allow wet feet to get cold. Even if they do not feel cold, dry them quickly and put on dry socks, in order to maintain body warmth.
- Do not use hot fomentations or poultices.

Shoes

Shoes must fit properly and provide adequate support. In fact, careful fitting and choice of shoes is probably the most important measure you can take to prevent foot problems.

- Wear comfortable, well-fitting shoes with soft uppers. Lace-ups with medium heels are ideal.
- Never accept shoes that you feel must be 'broken in'.
- When buying new shoes, always try them on, and rely on the advice of a qualified shoe fitter. Shoes must always be the correct shape for your feet.

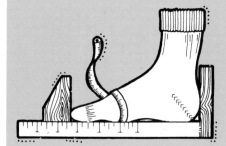

- Slippers do not provide adequate support. They should be worn only for short periods, and not throughout the day. Do not walk about in bare feet.
- Do not wear garters or socks with elasticated tops.

Daily rule Feel inside your shoes before putting them on. This is important, because you may not feel nails or pieces or grit under your feet, as a result of lost sensitivity in your feet.

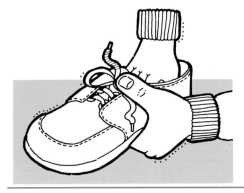

Corns and calluses

● Do not cut your corns and calluses yourself, or let a well-meaning friend cut them for you.

● Do not use corn paints or corn plasters. They contain acids which can be extremely dangerous to those with diabetes.

● Any corns, calluses, ingrowing nails, and other foot ailments should be treated by a State Registered Chiropodist.

First aid measures

● Minor injuries, such as cuts and abrasions, can be self-treated quite adequately by gently cleaning the area with soap and water and covering it with a sterile dressing.

● You should report to your doctor any injury that does not seem to be getting better within a couple of days.

● If blisters occur, do not prick them. If they burst, dress them as for a minor cut.

● Never use strong medicaments, such as iodine, Dettol, Germoline, or other powerful antiseptics.

● Never place adhesive strapping directly over a wound.

● If you are in the slightest doubt about how to deal with any wounds, discolourations, corns, and especially ulcers, consult your doctor or State Registered Chiropodist.

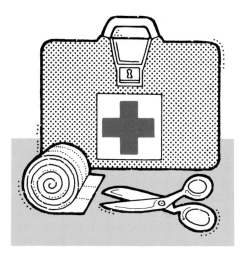

Damage to the eyes

Two parts of the eye are affected by diabetes.

1. **The lens**

   Opacities in the lens (cataracts) are common in elderly people, and may cause deterioration of vision. Cataracts occur more often in people with diabetes than in those who do not have it.

2. **The retina**

   This is the light-sensitive part of the back of the eye, which is responsible for transmitting visual images to the brain. Diabetes quite often causes minor abnormalities of the retina, without causing deterioration of vision – a condition described by the term 'diabetic retinopathy'. However, in a minority of sufferers, vision deteriorates, and without treatment the affected eye becomes blind, usually from bleeding (haemorrhage) within the eye.

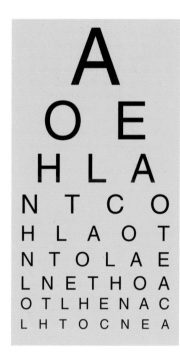

Prevention and treatment of eye damage

When cataracts seriously interfere with vision, they may be treated by surgery. You may be told when your eyes are examined that small cataracts are present. If you have no disturbance of vision do not be alarmed by this, as it is likely to be many years before treatment is necessary. When an operation is necessary, this is usually easily performed and a new lens inserted.

Fortunately, damage to the retina can now be treated and blindness prevented in many instances. Treatment is by laser, a process which involves aiming a fine beam of very bright light in the area of the diseased blood vessels. It is very simple to perform, but it has to be undertaken before sight has deteriorated too seriously.

Therefore, it is **essential** that you should have your eyes tested and the backs of your eyes examined regularly – ideally, annually. This can be done by an optician, by doctors in the clinic, or by an eye specialist.

Some blurring of vision may occur in the first few weeks of diabetes treatment. This is of no consequence and nearly always resolves within a few weeks – so do not get your glasses changed. Subsequently, if you should notice a sudden loss of vision in either eye, you **must** report it to your doctor immediately.

Contact lenses

People with diabetes should be aware that they have a higher risk of developing irritation of the eye from contact lens usage than those without diabetes. A meticulous cleaning routine and careful technique for lens handling is important. You should make sure you have been shown how to do this and you should have your technique checked from time to time. If you are using daily-wear soft lenses, these should be exchanged every six months.

Extended-wear soft lenses should not be generally prescribed for those with diabetes, as damage to the cornea is more common with this type. If your eyes become red or irritated, you should immediately stop using contact lenses and seek advice.

Damage to the kidneys

Damage to the kidneys occurs less frequently than eye damage. Kidney damage must be present for many years before function begins to deteriorate, and then a few more years usually elapse before the situation becomes serious. Unfortunately, there are no symptoms relating to kidney disease until it is quite advanced. However, regular checks of your urine will reveal early changes, which should enable steps to be taken to avoid further deterioration.

Painful neuritis

Rarely, neuritis causes pain, usually in the feet and legs, which is particularly disagreeable. A burning sensation, a feeling of pins-and-needles, and an excruciating discomfort on contact with clothes or bedclothes are the main characteristics of this condition. These symptoms can be very unpleasant, but they usually disappear in time, although it may take many months for them to do so. Very good control is an essential part of treatment, and this often requires the use of insulin. Various tablets, including painkillers, are also used in treating this condition.

Impotence

Sometimes nerve damage causes impotence. It should be remembered, however, that impotence is also common in those without diabetes. It is often due to psychological causes. Short periods (weeks or months) of impotence are common, especially in middle-aged men, during periods of stress. In the great majority, the problem is only temporary and they recover. Proper diagnosis is important, so do not hesitate to ask for advice. Treatment is now available for many, including special counselling and certain devices designed to overcome the problem. In severe cases, a specific injection therapy works very well. Diabetes specialists are very aware of these problems, so do not be embarrassed to ask if you have been having difficulties.

Arterial disease

Hardening and narrowing of the arteries are normal consequences of ageing, but with diabetes there may be slight acceleration of this process. Arterial disease can result in heart attacks, and cause poor circulation in the feet and legs. Keeping to your recommended diet will help to reduce your risk of arterial disease.

Diabetes and other illnesses

Treatment for these disorders is exactly the same as in those without diabetes. You should take the following precautions to keep the risk of arterial disease to a minimum

- Do not smoke
- Do not become overweight
- Have your blood pressure checked annually and treated if necessary
- Reduce the amount of fat in your diet
- Take as much exercise as you can.

The effect of illness on diabetes

In the section on the effectiveness of your treatment (Chapter 5) it was indicated that under certain circumstances your diabetes may go temporarily out of control. Although a few days' loss of control is of no real significance, if you should develop symptoms of **thirst** and **dryness of the mouth** or **pass large quantities of urine**, you should consult your doctor.

Associated illnesses

Very occasionally, diabetes may be associated with another illness, or it may actually be part of another illness. Sometimes diabetes apparently develops as a result of the treatment given for other illnesses. Disorders of the liver and pancreas, excess iron stores in the body, and hormonal problems involving the thyroid and adrenal glands are quite often associated with diabetes. Generally, such problems will be identified when you first see your doctor. Treatment will be prescribed in parallel with the treatment for your diabetes.

Diabetes and the treatment of other illnesses

Diabetes is no bar to the treatment (including operations) of any other disorder or illness. Because your diabetes may not be so easily controlled during a period of sickness, your diabetes treatment may need temporary adjustment.

Certain drugs cause a rise in blood sugar (e.g. steroids and water tablets). It may be suggested that you change these. Alternatively, your doctor may advise an increase in treatment for your diabetes.

Dentistry

Straightforward, routine dental treatment can be carried out by your dentist in the normal way. When the treatment involves general anaesthesia, however, then this should always be performed by a hospital team and not in the dental surgery.

Diabetic control whilst in hospital

When you are in hospital you are usually confined to bed and will not be taking any exercise. You may be anxious, and your diet will most probably be different. Together these factors will undoubtedly cause your blood tests to become raised. Consequently, your diabetes treatment will need to be increased. Tablets may be introduced for the first time, or their dose increased. Sometimes insulin will be recommended, almost always on a temporary basis. You should realize that the cause of these changes in your diabetic control is the result of prevailing circumstances, and **not** a failure on your part or on the part of the hospital staff.

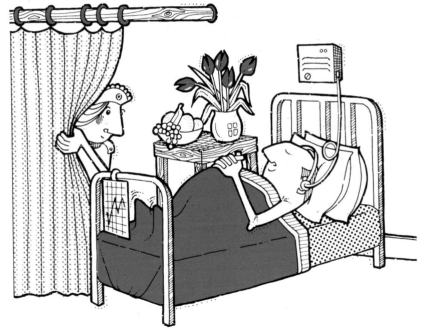

Clinic attendance

Regular medical check-ups

OUTPATIENT APPOINTMENTS

Name _____

Address _____

_____

Date	Time	Consultant	Clinic

Bring this card with you to the hospital

The organization of clinics

Your local diabetic clinic plays an important role in the treatment and control of your diabetes. The organization of these clinics varies in different areas of the country. In the majority of cases it is at the local hospital and is under the direction of a hospital consultant. Many units have set up special diabetes centres with expertly trained doctors, nurses, dietitians, and chiropodists. In many districts clinics have been established in specially-trained general practices, or co-operative schemes have been developed between hospital specialists and family doctors. Evening clinics may be held to enable you to attend after work.

In the period after your diabetes has been diagnosed, your doctor may wish to see you every few weeks, until he or she is sure that the treatment is effective. However, when your blood sugar has been brought under control, your doctor may want to see you perhaps only every few months or, if you are very well controlled, yearly.

With your urine or blood test records you will be able to keep a routine check on the effectiveness of your treatment. None the less, from time to time it is **essential** that you visit your doctor or clinic so that your treatment can be monitored, and any specific problems you might have can be dealt with.

● Your doctor will want to be sure that your tests are satisfactory. If the record of your tests shows erratic or high sugar levels, he or she will decide whether additional treatment is necessary.

● Your doctor will want to perform a blood test to check your control, because sometimes your own tests may be misleading.

● Your doctor will want to ensure that you understand and are happy with the advice you have been given. This is the time for you to ask questions!

● From time to time, your doctor will want to check whether any long-term complications have developed. It is important that these should be detected before you notice anything wrong, so that early treatment can be commenced.

● Finally, such visits provide you with an opportunity to discuss problems with, for example, your dietitian. You should also report any new symptoms, such as difficulty with vision or problems with your feet.

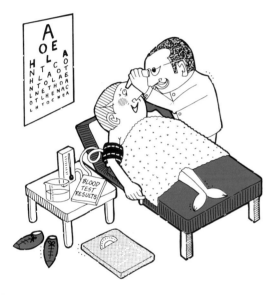

We recommend that once your diabetes is reasonably controlled you should do the following.

1. See a specialist nurse, doctor, dietitian and chiropodist at regular intervals – annually, or more often if necessary. These meetings should give time for discussion as well as for assessing your control.

2. Be able to contact any member of the health care team for specialist advice when you need it.

3. Have more education sessions as you are ready for them.

4. Have a formal medical review once a year by a doctor experienced in diabetes.

   At this review the following should happen.

   ● Your weight should be recorded.
   ● Your urine should be tested for ketones and protein.
   ● Your blood should be tested to measure long-term control.
   ● You should discuss control, including your home monitoring results.
   ● Your blood pressure should be checked.
   ● Your vision should be checked, and the back of your eyes examined with an ophthalmoscope. If necessary you should be referred to an ophthalmologist.
   ● Your legs and feet should be examined to check your circulation and nerve supply. If necessary you should be referred to a chiropodist.
   ● Your injection sites should be examined if you are on insulin.
   ● You should have the opportunity to discuss how you are coping at home and at work.

The control of your diabetes is important, and so is the detection and treatment of any complications. Make sure you are getting the medical care and education you need to ensure you stay healthy. If you are not feeling well, or if your treatment appears not be working, or if you develop any unusual symptoms such as worsening eyesight, or abnormal tingling in the hands or feet, report to your doctor at once – **DO NOT WAIT FOR YOUR NEXT APPOINTMENT.**

Summary

It must be stressed that the problems of long-term diabetes occur only in a minority of people with diabetes.

Remember

- Good control of diabetes usually prevents the development of these complications. Therefore, advice from regular clinic attendance is very important.
- Smoking accelerates arterial disease (affecting the heart and feet), and may also have a bad effect on your eyes and kidneys.
- Try and control your weight.
- Keep a regular eye on your own tests.

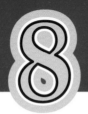

Diabetes and your daily life

This chapter answers some of the most frequently asked questions about the influence of diabetes on your everyday activities. It discusses topics such as the financial implications of diabetes, and the additional steps you may need to take in order to remain fit and active.

Non-insulin dependent diabetes is, in the majority of cases, easily controlled by diet, or by diet and tablets, and should therefore make very little difference to your daily life. Undoubtedly, the greatest change will be the need to modify and regulate your diet, but other day-to-day activities should need to be altered very little.

Employment

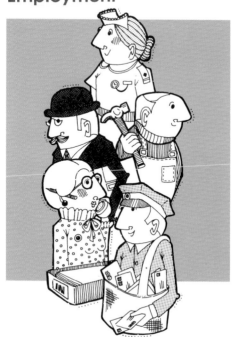

Diabetes and its influence on your work

For the vast majority of those with non-insulin dependent diabetes, their condition has no effect on their work. Consequently, your ability to function well should be as good as before you developed diabetes, perhaps even better. There are certain careers in which having diabetes can prove a hindrance.

● If your work involves driving a passenger carrying vehicle, and you have to take tablets for the treatment of your diabetes, then certain restrictions may be imposed.

● Because of statutory regulations, you will not be allowed to fly aeroplanes.

● In some occupations, employers impose rather strict health regulations. For example, you cannot be accepted for entry into the armed services, the police, or the fire service, although if you are an established member you should be able to continue without difficulty.

● If you have a potentially highly dangerous job, e.g. deep-sea diving, steeplejacking, or any job for which very high standards of fitness are required, you will probably have to change your occupation.

Diabetes and your employer

Unless you work in one of the occupations mentioned above, your employer need have no fears about your ability to continue employment or commence a new job. Unfortunately, some employers do not know very much about diabetes and are therefore often reluctant to employ anybody with diabetes, in the mistaken belief that they might prove to be an unreliable employee. Therefore, you should stress to your employer that with uncomplicated diabetes you are as capable of performing your job as a person without diabetes, and without risk to yourself or others. Shift work should pose no problems and, unlike those with insulin dependent diabetes, you do not require specific breaks for snacks or additional meals.

Occasionally, employers will not employ people with diabetes, because of their fear of future problems. In particular, they may be apprehensive that late complications may develop and render an employee incapable of full-time work.

If you experience difficulty in convincing your employer that you are fit to take up a new job, or to continue in your existing one, enlist the help of your family doctor or hospital doctor and, if necessary, the British Diabetic Association.

Only rarely should a person with diabetes need to be registered as disabled with the Disablement Resettlement Officer at the local job centre. However, should you develop serious complications, particularly loss of vision, you may find it helpful to register, and should not consider it a stigma to do so.

Financial implications of having diabetes

Insurance

Having diabetes should not give rise to any serious financial problems. Where you may experience some increased expenditure, however, is in the field of life insurance. In **all** matters relating to insurance, it is essential to be **completely** frank with brokers or insurers. Concealment of any important medical facts may invalidate the insurance offered, with potentially serious financial and legal consequences. There is no need, however, to inform your insurance company of your diabetes for any life policies taken out **before** your diagnosis.

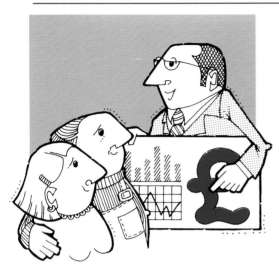

Motor insurance

If you hold a motor insurance policy, you **must** notify your insurance company or insurance broker **immediately** that you develop diabetes. Failure to do so may cause liability to be denied in the event of a claim. Most insurance companies will continue to offer cover to clients who develop diabetes. Some companies may require a medical certificate from your doctor. Attempts to impose an additional premium because of the diabetes should be resisted.

New applicants for motor insurance may experience problems, but certain companies will quote normal rates, provided no accidents related to diabetes have occurred (there should be none in your case). If you encounter difficulties, details of the BDA's broker may be obtained from the British Diabetic Association.

Life insurance

Because of the possibility of long-term complications developing, it is normal for some loading to be placed on life and health insurance policies. If your diabetes is perfectly controlled and you have no complications, this loading should be small or non-existent, but may be 5–10 per cent on whole life policies. Loading for term assurance, e.g. mortgage protection or endowment policies, will be higher, but will normally be less than for those who are treated with insulin. If you experience any problems, you should seek help from the British Diabetic Association.

Sickness, accident and holiday insurance

It is **essential** that you declare your diabetes when taking out life or health insurance. Those with diabetes seeking personal sickness and accident insurance are likely to have to pay higher than normal premiums.

Those taking out insurance in connection with travel and holidays abroad must pay particular attention to the exclusion clauses. They normally exclude all pre-existing illnesses, i.e. those present before you travel. However, special cover for people with diabetes can usually be arranged, and the British Diabetic Association can give advice on this matter. Do not forget that failing to declare your diabetes when taking out travel insurance could nullify the policy.

Pensions and superannuation

Your pension rights should be unaffected by your diabetes. If you enter into a new scheme, it is essential that you declare your diabetes.

Other financial considerations

- Prescription charges in the UK are waived for people with diabetes treated with tablets and insulin, but not if the diabetes is treated by diet alone. A form (AB11), available from your family doctor, or Social Security office, gives details of prescription exemption, so that you may obtain an exemption certificate. This applies to all prescriptions, whether related to your diabetes or not. People with diabetes are also entitled to free eye tests.
- Some people may find that they have to spend more money on buying a healthy diet, and on such items as suitable footwear. If you are dependent on Social Security for your income, it may be worthwhile contacting your local Citizens Advice Bureau or Welfare Rights Service to make sure that you are getting your full entitlement.
- Those who develop late complications, especially with their eyes, may be eligible for additional benefits.
- The BDA has a leaflet on Social Security and Social Services. There are no special provisions which especially apply to people with diabetes, but the leaflet gives information on the financial and practical help which is generally available.

Points to remember

You must

- Tell your insurance company that you have diabetes.
- Tell the licensing authorities (Drivers Medical Branch, DVLC, Swansea SA99 1TU) that you have diabetes.

Applying for a driving licence

When you apply for a driving licence you have to answer a question on whether you have diabetes.

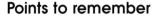

Driving

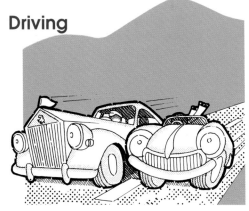

To this question you should answer 'Yes', whether you have diabetes treated with insulin, or diet and tablets, or diet alone. In the space provided for details, you should state that you have diabetes, adding that your diabetes is controlled by diet, diet and tablets, or insulin, as appropriate.

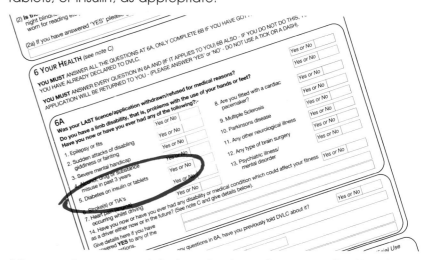

Fig. 8.1
Driving licence application
It is important to answer the question regarding diabetes correctly.

After you have completed and returned your application form, you may be sent another form, asking for further information. This will include the name and address of your doctor or hospital clinic, as well as your consent for the Driver and Vehicle Licensing Centre to approach your doctor for a detailed report on your diabetes. This complication of procedure does not mean that you will be refused a driving licence. The licence will normally be issued without delay for three years and renewals will be made free of charge.

If your diabetes was diagnosed only recently and you already hold a 'life' licence, this will be revoked and replaced with a 'period' licence. Renewals can take several weeks, but should your licence pass its expiry date, you can continue to drive **providing** you have made application for a renewal. Heavy goods vehicle (HGV) licences and passenger carrying vehicle (PCV) licences are not prohibited to those with diabetes who do not take insulin, although some restrictions may be imposed on the public service vehicle driver.

If you have non-insulin dependent diabetes controlled by diet alone, and have normal eyesight (with glasses if necessary), there are no special precautions which you need take.

If, however, you take tablets you

● Must ensure that you have your meals regularly

● Should not drive if you are already late for a meal.

If you have any problems obtaining a driving licence, you should contact the British Diabetic Association.

Exercise and sport

Exercise is an important aspect of the overall programme to control your diabetes. It not only lowers your blood sugar, but makes the action of insulin on your fat and muscle cells more efficient. Therefore, exercise is very beneficial and is actively encouraged. There is no reason why you should not be able to continue heavy manual work, or continue to enjoy any of the sports you played before your diabetes was diagnosed. There are leading tennis and badminton players, golfers, swimmers, cricketers, athletes, and professional footballers who have diabetes.

Unlike a person with insulin dependent diabetes, there is usually no need for you to adjust your diet before strenuous exercise. If you are taking tablets, however, your blood sugar may fall lower than usual during exercise. This can be readily put right by an extra snack of carbohydrate-containing food.

If you are a more sedentary type of person, not given to playing sport, you should, if possible, take routine, moderate exercise. Regular walking, for example, is better than short bursts of very strenuous exercise, and it can do much to preserve and even improve the circulation. Although a great deal of such mild exercise may be needed to reduce weight, it can make a contribution towards this goal. Keeping fit is an essential aspect of maintaining good diabetic control.

Fig. 8.2
Keeping fit is an essential aspect of
maintaining good diabetic control

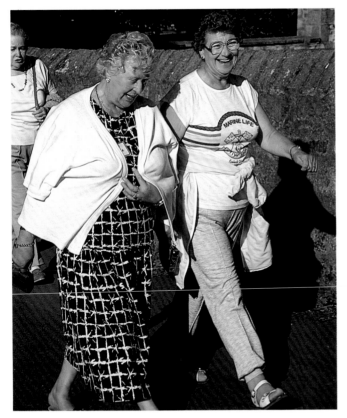

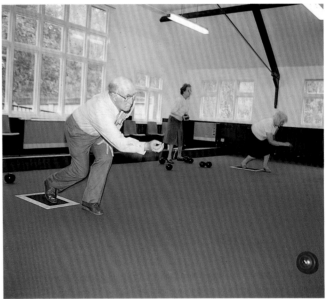

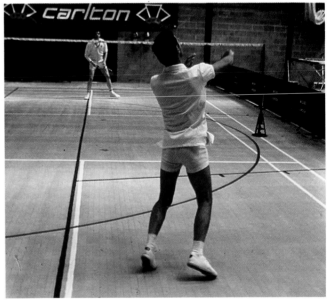

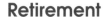

Retirement

All retired people have to adjust to stopping the normal routine of going to work, and to the fact that they are no longer associating with colleagues and workmates. Loss of such contacts and interests may lead to bouts of depression, particularly in those who have never developed hobbies or interests outside their work. However, as long as you are otherwise fit, retirement should cause no greater problems for you than for anybody else.

If you are retired, it is essential that you should not allow your diabetes to stop you from developing new interests, or from making an active contribution to the community. For example, you could undertake voluntary work for the British Diabetic Association or other charitable organizations.

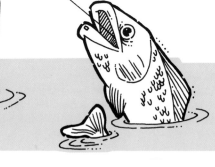

Do not forget to take advantage of the various benefits available to you as a retired person. Reduced fares on public transport and reduced entrance fees to certain places of entertainment, for example, could provide you with many opportunities not previously enjoyed.

Maintaining careful control of your diabetes, and taking whatever exercise is possible, are the best ways to ensuring that you remain healthy into old age.

Remember to ask your doctor or dietitian about adjustments to your diet if your activity level increases or decreases.

Fig. 8.3
Do not let your diabetes stop you
from enjoying a full and active
retirement

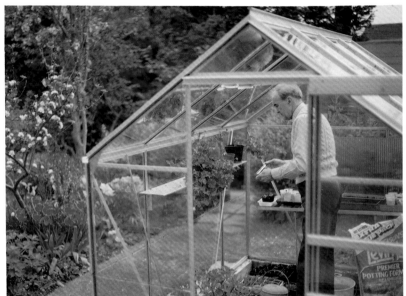

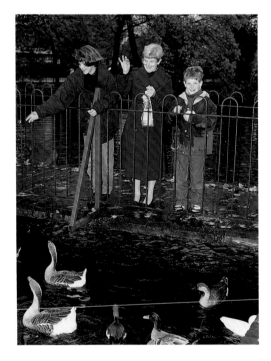

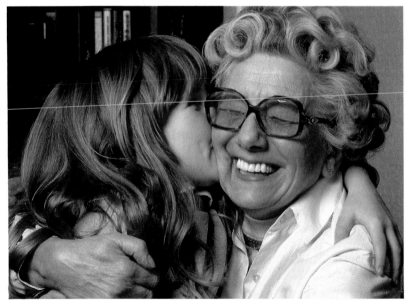

Travel and holidays

Your form of diabetes should not impose restrictions on travelling or holidays. It is wise, however, to take certain essential precautions, bearing in mind that even people without diabetes frequently suffer unforseen circumstances away from home.

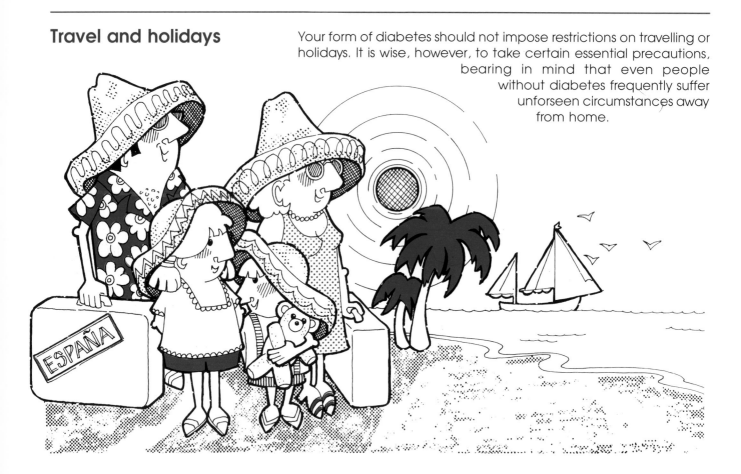

Illness

Mild gastroenteritis is an ailment commonly suffered while travelling abroad, and could cause your diabetes to go temporarily out of control.

Whenever you feel unwell whilst travelling, test your urine or blood sugar. If the results show a high sugar reading, and you feel very dry and thirsty, consult a doctor. Most of the illnesses you are likely to experience while away from home will be mild and of short duration. All you may notice are positive urine tests or high blood tests for a day or so, which then return to normal.

These are the most important points to remember when travelling at home or abroad.

- Take your diabetes testing equipment with you.
- If you take tablets, carry more than you are likely to require. This is particularly important when travelling abroad, in case your return should be delayed.
- When travelling overseas, always take out health insurance.
- Always carry a card indicating that you have diabetes – this is essential if you take tablets.

Fig. 8.4
Always carry some form of identification

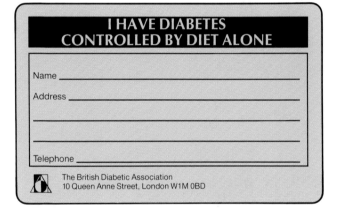

**I HAVE DIABETES
CONTROLLED BY TABLETS**

Name _____

Address _____

_____

Telephone _____

If I am found ill, please give me 2 teaspoons of sugar in a small amount of water or 3 glucose tablets which I am carrying.
If I fail to recover in 10 minutes, please call an ambulance (Dial 999).
   The British Diabetic Association
   10 Queen Anne Street, London W1M 0BD

**I HAVE DIABETES
CONTROLLED BY DIET ALONE**

Name _____

Address _____

_____

_____

Telephone _____

   The British Diabetic Association
   10 Queen Anne Street, London W1M 0BD

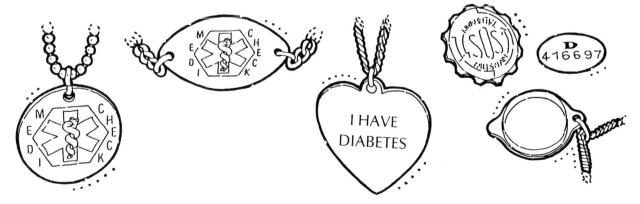

Contraception, pregnancy and parenthood

Foreign food

Eating different food, cooked in an unfamiliar way, may cause some problems, especially when eating out. Usually, though, you will find little difficulty in recognizing food similar to that of your normal diet.

An occasional deviation from your normal diet will do no harm, and may merely cause an isolated positive urine test or high blood test. If, however, you are overweight and have been on a diet, do not spoil all your previous good work.

Air travel

You are not subject to any special restrictions, and you need take no special precautions.

Vaccinations

Diabetes does not impose any restrictions on the vaccinations you may need if travelling abroad. However, immunisation against certain illnesses may be followed by a day or so of feeling mildly unwell, together with a temporary rise in your blood sugar. This should cause you no concern.

Travel guides

Travel guides for many of the popular tourist destinations are available from the BDA. Contact the BDA for further information.

Contraception

Because non-insulin dependent diabetes usually occurs in women who are middle-aged, contraception may not be a matter of concern. If, however, you are of an appropriate age, then you should seek advice on contraception from your doctor or family planning clinic. Although the risk to a woman's health from the normal contraceptive pill is very slight, in your case your diabetes may increase this risk slightly. The contraceptive pill may also lead to a rise in blood sugar, in which case some other form of contraception may be advisable.

Fig. 8.5
Diabetes should not prevent you from getting married and having a family

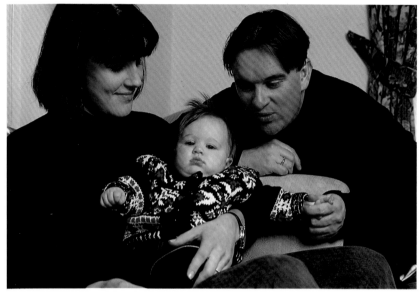

Pregnancy

If you are of child-bearing age and you intend having a child, there are two very important things you should do.

1. You must ensure that your diabetes is well controlled when you are **planning** the pregnancy.

2. It is **absolutely essential** that, once you know you are pregnant, you achieve perfect control and maintain it throughout pregnancy. The reason for this is that your growing baby, even though it will not have diabetes, will be subject to your insulin and blood sugar levels.

Therefore, if you are planning a pregnancy, and certainly as soon as you become pregnant, you must contact your doctor and/or hospital clinic. Also, in order to make sure that your pregnancy continues without problems, you must regularly attend your diabetic clinic.

You may find that you require additional treatment during pregnancy, or even a period in hospital. Such special measures can usually be stopped as soon as the baby has been delivered. With care by yourself and your doctor, a successful outcome is the rule.

Diabetes and heredity

The question asked by most parents is: 'What are the chances of my child having diabetes?' There is no easy answer to this question, because the way in which diabetes is inherited is a complex process, which is not yet fully understood. In non-insulin dependent diabetes it does appear that inheritance plays a more significant role than in insulin dependent diabetes. It must be stressed that it is most unlikely that any of your children will develop diabetes during childhood, as most inherited diabetes develops only later in life.

Many people who inherit the tendency to develop diabetes never actually do so. This is because other factors, including damage to the pancreas, emotional factors, obesity, and, in some instances even virus infections, are necessary for the development of diabetes.

Effect on the family

When you are first told that you have diabetes, a chronic lifelong condition, you may well feel confused and upset. This is a very normal reaction and you may find that your family feel equally worried by the diagnosis. Talking about these feelings with each other, with the health professionals involved in your diabetes care, and with other people with diabetes and their families can help.

With time, the majority of people come to terms with their diabetes, as they learn more about it. This learning about diabetes is recognized as a very important part of the treatment. Equally important is keeping your family up to date with this information. Most clinics will encourage you to bring someone with you for educational sessions. The people around you will be more able to give you the help and support you need to live with your diabetes, if they have the same information as you.

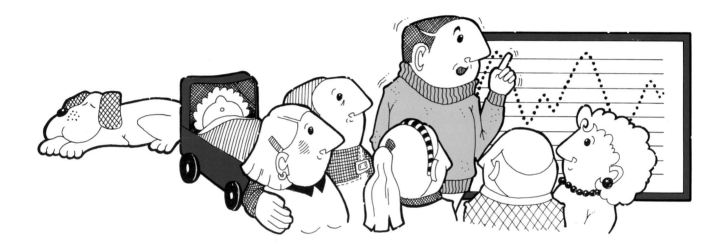

If the members of your family want to understand more about diabetes, the local group of the BDA can also be very helpful, and membership is open to the whole family.

Who is available to help?

With diet and tablets you should be able to control your diabetes. From time to time, however, you may develop problems about which you need specialist advice. On such occasions you may refer to a variety of individuals, including your doctor, nurses, dietitians, chiropodists, the Social Services and, of course, your local hospital clinic.

In the next chapter we also describe the help available to you from the BDA.

Some final comments on diabetes and your everyday life

- With relatively straightforward modifications to your daily life, effective control of your blood sugar level is possible.
- Stick to your diet.
- If you have managed to lose weight, do not put it on again!
- If you need to take tablets, take them regularly.
- Take reasonable care of your general health, and your feet in particular.
- Attend your clinic for regular check-ups.

The late Dr. R. D. Lawrence, physician and co-founder of the British Diabetic Association, wrote in his famous book *The Diabetic Life:*

'There is no reason why a diabetic should not, if he can be taught to do so, lead a long and normal life. True, the diabetic life demands self-control from all its subjects, but it gives in return a full and active existence, with no real privations.'

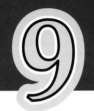

The British Diabetic Association

This chapter describes the work of the British Diabetic Association and how it may be of help to you.

The BDA was founded in 1934 and provides information and advice on all aspects of diabetes. The BDA also acts as your representative, campaigning for better services and to overcome public ignorance and prejudice.

The Association supports research to improve treatments and to find a cure or means of prevention for diabetes and its problems.

The Association depends entirely upon voluntary subscriptions and donations and needs your support. The more members we have, the greater our influence on your behalf.

How the BDA helps support those with diabetes

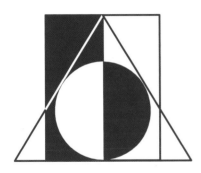

Liaison with other bodies

The BDA is in close contact with other professional bodies and also with the media. One of the Association's aims is to ensure that diabetes is portrayed correctly and kept in the public eye, thereby helping to eliminate prejudice.

The Association also maintains close contact with government departments and other voluntary organizations to ensure a mutual exchange of information. The Association has been extremely successful in its campaigns to obtain medical equipment on general prescription for people with diabetes.

The BDA has an important role in ensuring that standards of diabetes health care are maintained and monitored. Its reports and recommendations on different aspects of care are recognized nationally and adopted at a local level.

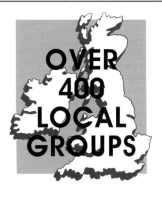

Nationwide organization

In the UK there are over 400 local groups, which hold regular meetings, and all branches welcome new members. Through your local branch you will be able to meet other people with diabetes, and talk about the everyday aspects of living with diabetes. Details of your nearest local branch will be sent to you when you join the Association, or alternatively you can ring the Head Office for details.

General information

The BDA can provide guidance and help on all issues affecting those with diabetes. However, it is not able to give advice on individual medical treatment, as this must come from your own medical carers. The BDA answers several thousand telephone calls and letters every month, on a wide variety of different topics. It is able to give general dietary advice, suggestions for recipes and slimming ideas, as well as information on all the practical aspects of life, such as diabetes equipment, car driving, insurance, travelling abroad, etc.

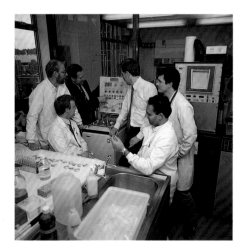

Research

One of the most important aspects of the BDA's work is research. The Association is the UK's largest single contributor to diabetic research in hospitals and universities, and currently supports over 60 grants, totalling well over £2 million each year.

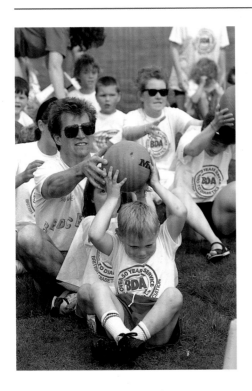

Holidays for young people with diabetes

The Youth Department runs educational and activity holidays for children and teenagers with diabetes. This gives them the opportunity to learn about their diabetes whilst taking part in activities, without being the 'odd one out'. In addition, family weekends, parents meetings, and international exchanges are organized. Pen-pals can also be put in touch with each other.

Balance: a bi-monthly magazine

Members receive *Balance*, the magazine of the BDA, free of charge, every two months. It reports progress in medical care, and the latest news on legislation that affects those with diabetes. There is information on healthy eating and recipes, articles on personalities, and practical hints on day-to-day living.

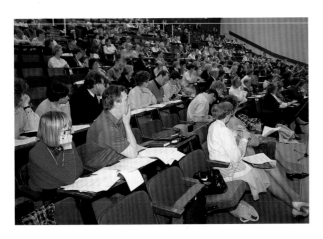

Conferences on diabetes

Through the Medical and Scientific, Education, and Professional Services Sections of the Association, conferences and study days are organized for all health care professionals concerned with diabetes, to ensure that they are kept up to date with advances in care and treatment. The BDA is continually striving to make the life of people with diabetes easier and better in every way.

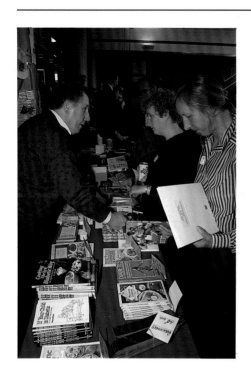

Publications

The BDA produces a wide range of publications on diabetes including books, leaflets, information sheets, posters, and videos. For a comprehensive list of publications, please ask the BDA to send you their latest catalogue and order form.

The address is

> British Diabetic Association
> 10 Queen Anne Street
> London W1M OBD

The telephone number is

> 071 323 1531.

The BDA is a registered charity, number 215199.

A charity helping people with diabetes and supporting diabetes research

 BRITISH DIABETIC ASSOCIATION

Index

insulin treatment
in insulin dependent diabetes 4, 8
in non-insulin dependent diabetes 4,
20, 63-68
temporary 62, 65, 77
insulin-producing cells 3, 4-5, 12
insurance 66, 82-83, 91
islets of Langerhans 3, 4-5, 12
itching, of the genitals 6, 16

J

jobs *see* work
juvenile diabetes *see* insulin dependent
diabetes

K

kidney damage 75
kilocalories *see* calories
kilojoules 22

L

lens of the eye 73
life insurance 83
liver 2, 11, 12, 76
long-term effects of diabetes 17, 52
on arteries 19, 75
on eyes 73
on feet 69
on kidneys 69, 75
on nerves 69, 75
prevention of 2, 19, 69
and social security benefits 84

M

maturity onset diabetes *see* non-insulin
dependent diabetes
meals
eating regularly 20, 42, 66
effect on blood sugar levels 2, 11, 13,
63-64
meals *continued*

foreign food 92
menu suggestions 43-49
see also diet; food; snacks
meat 25, 34, 35
medical check-ups 78-79
medical review, annual 79
medication *see* drugs; tablet treatment
metabolism 9-10
meters, blood glucose 59-60
metformin 51, 54
minerals 26
monounsaturated fats 25-26
motor insurance 66, 83, 84

N

needles 63
neuritis 69, 75
neuropathy *see* neuritis
non-insulin dependent diabetes 3
diet treatment 4, 19-50
effect on blood sugar levels 12, 13
heredity 4, 6, 15, 94
insulin treatment 4, 63-68
long-term effects 69-76
loss of control 61-62
symptomless 5, 7, 17, 55
symptoms 6-7, 15-17
tablet treatment 51-54
what causes it 4, 14
who gets it 14-15
normoglycaemia 14

O

overweight
  causes 11, 22
  effect on blood cholesterol 26
  effect on insulin activity 12, 15, 20, 66
  increased chances of developing non-insulin dependent diabetes 4, 15
  weight chart 41
  see also dieting to lose weight

P

painful neuritis 75
pancreas 3, 12
  diseases of 5, 76
  not producing enough insulin 13, 14, 15
  reaction to changes in blood sugar levels 11, 13
  tablets which stimulate insulin production in 51
pasta 22, 23, 27
pastry 21, 25, 31, 34, 35
PCV licences 81, 85
pensions 84
polyunsaturated fats 25-26
pregnancy 65, 93
prescription charges 84
prevention
  of arterial disease 19, 76
  of bowel problems 23
  of complications 2, 19, 69
  of eye damage 74
  of foot problems 70-73
  of hypoglycaemia 64, 66
protein 21, 25
  metabolism 9-10
pulses 22, 23, 25, 28

R

records
  blood tests 60
  urine tests 58
renal threshold 14, 56
retina 73, 74
retinopathy, diabetic 73
retirement 88-89
rice 23, 27, 28
roughage *see* fibre

S

salt 36
saturated fats 25-26
shoes 69, 72
sickness insurance 83
smoking 70, 76, 80
snacks 66
  during exercise 86
  effect on blood sugar levels 2, 11, 63-64
  see also diet; food; meals
social security 84
soluble fibre 23, 24, 28
sport *see* exercise
starch splitters 54
starchy foods 11, 22-23
stress 12, 15, 57, 61
sugar
  alternatives to 32-33
  in baking 33
  controlling intake of 20, 22, 27, 31-32, 66
  see also blood sugar
superannuation 84
sweeteners, artificial 32-33

W

weakness 16

weighing, regular 61

weight chart 41

weight loss

    deliberate *see* dieting to lose weight

    symptom of diabetes 6, 16, 61

work 81-82

    jobs imposing restrictions 67, 81

    when on insulin treatment 66, 67

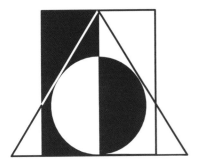

THE BRITISH DIABETIC ASSOCIATION

offers you a welcome

MEMBERSHIP ENROLMENT FORM

Please fill in all sections of the form (Use BLOCK LETTERS)
This information will be treated as strictly confidential.

Title _____ Forename(s) _____

Surname _____

Address _____

_____

_____

Post Code _____

Telephone No. _____

Occupation _____ Date of Birth _____

Sex   Male ☐   Female ☐

Tear off and return

Tick a box to indicate the type of membership you require:

☐ **Annual Member:**   **£10.00 a year**

☐ **Family Member:**   **£12.50 a year**
(You will be sent a form asking for additional information about any members of your family who have diabetes)

☐ **Reduced Rate:**   **£2.00 a year**
(Please indicate whether you are: pensioner/student on a Government grant/in receipt of a DSS benefit)

☐ **Life Member:**   **£175.00**
(£25 a year for 7 years under covenant. Covenant forms available on request)

☐ **Are you joining on behalf of a child?**
(Children in the UK under the age of 18 can join free for one year if they wish)

☐ **Overseas Annual Member:**   **£20.00 a year**

☐ **Overseas Life Member:**   **£200.00**

I enclose my cheque ☐ postal order ☐ banker's order ☐

for £ _____   payable to the British Diabetic Association

or debit my (please tick box) ACCESS ☐   VISA ☐

Credit card number _____ or
Giro Account No. 53 430 0006

Card Expiry Date _____

BANKER'S ORDER FORM

To _____ Bank,

Address _____ Branch _____

Please pay to the National Westminster Bank Limited, 154 Harley Street, London W1N 2AS (60.10.02)

the sum of £ _____ (words _____

) on the _____ day of _____ 19__

and a like sum annually on the same date until further notice for the credit of the British Diabetic Association (A/c no. 12773085)

A/c no _____

Signed _____

Name (BLOCK CAPITALS) _____

Address _____

After completing the above form, please return to THE ACCOUNTANT, BRITISH DIABETIC ASSOCIATION 10 QUEEN ANNE STREET, LONDON W1M 0BD

Do you have diabetes?　YES ☐　NO ☐

If so, please fill in the following information:

Types of diabetes:

Insulin Dependent (Type I) ☐　　Non-Insulin Dependent (Type II) ☐

Date of Diagnosis ☐

If you are taking insulin what method of treatment are you using?

Human Insulin: ☐　　Animal Insulin:　Pork ☐　　Beef ☐

Have you taken insulin from diagnosis?　YES ☐　　NO ☐

If you are not taking insulin what method of treatment are you using?

Tablets and Diet ☐　　Diet Alone ☐

How did you hear about the BDA?

BDA Branch ☐　　Clinic ☐　　Hospital ☐

Magazine ☐　　Friend ☐

Other (please specify)
☐

Would you like your name forwarded to your local branch?

YES ☐　　NO ☐

Signature _____　　Date _____

FOR OFFICE USE ONLY

Please return your completed form to:
BRITISH DIABETIC ASSOCIATION, 10 QUEEN ANNE STREET,
LONDON, W1M 0BD. (TEL. NO: 071-323 1531)

The BDA invites you to:

■ *Become a member.* The Enrolment Form lists the different types of membership. Fill it in and return it to the BDA.
If you want your annual subscription to be paid regularly by your bank with no further fuss, please complete the Bankers Order Form and send it to the BDA.

■ *Remember the BDA in your will.* Legacies are all-important to the Association. A legacy, however small, will be a valuable contribution to the BDA research programme.

■ *Send us a donation.* We rely very much on the generosity of donors. If you wish to donate regularly, please take advantage of some tax concessions. Three of these are listed below – (a) tax efficient to us, (b) tax efficient to you and (c) tax efficient to both of us.

a) Deed of Covenant: If you expect to be paying income tax for more than the next three years, please ask for a Deed of Covenant form. A Deed of Covenant means we can recover the basic rate of tax you have already paid. That's an extra 25% or more for the BDA's work.

b) Payroll giving: If you are employed and pay tax, you can donate any amount up to a total of £600 per year. As this amount is deducted from you gross pay and is tax-free, your donation costs you less. Your employer should be able to tell you about this scheme.

c) Gift Aid: If you can give £600 or more and pay tax, please give through the Gift Aid Scheme. We will supply you with a form.

Notes

Notes